Hypnotism

Psychology and Hypnosis Driven
Sales Closing Techinques

*(The Ultimate Guide to Neuro Linguistic
Programming Training and Hypnotherapy)*

Diana Daniels

Published By **Zoe Lawson**

Diana Daniels

Hypnotism: Psychology and Hypnosis Driven Sales Closing Techinques (The Ultimate Guide to Neuro Linguistic Programming Training and Hypnotherapy)

ISBN 978-1-998901-51-7

No part of this guidebook shall be reproduced in any form without permission in writing from the publisher except in the case of brief quotations embodied in critical articles or reviews.

Legal & Disclaimer

The information contained in this ebook is not designed to replace or take the place of any form of medicine or professional medical advice. The information in this ebook has been provided for educational & entertainment purposes only.

The information contained in this book has been compiled from sources deemed reliable, and it is accurate to the best of the Author's knowledge; however, the Author cannot guarantee its accuracy and validity and cannot be held liable for any errors or omissions. Changes are periodically made to this book. You must consult your doctor or get professional medical advice before using any of the suggested remedies, techniques, or information in this book.

Table Of Contents

Chapter 1: What is Hypnosis?

When you think of the idea of hypnosis, you might visualize a mysterious figure who could swing an electronic watch in front of your eyes. After that, you might believe that anyone who is under hypnosis will follow whatever the hypnotist commands him to do like they've been able to create a master-slave partnership within an instant. However, hypnosis goes deeper than this popular mythology.

Hypnosis Defined

Hypnosis is the method that allows you to enter into the state of consciousness in which you let the portion of your brain responsible the subconscious mind to control your thinking process. In other words, when you're hypnotized you stimulate the right portion of your brain that is responsible for your autopilot actions, creativity and imagination.

Hypnosis can also make you vulnerable to influence and suggestions because you're suppressing that part of the brain that controls logic, you're in a position to shift your assumptions about what you are able to accomplish. This technique allows you to suggest ideas, let your mind let forgotten memories to come back into focus, or aid you in changing your habits.

Due to this it is an extremely controversial method due to the fact that it makes an individual think about things that they normally avoid even consider. To the point where it could cause a person to into doing things that appear be out of his control Some people consider this method as a risky one.

A deeper understanding of what happens when you are hypnotized will help you realize what could occur under a hypnotic trance and to what extent is it possible for a person to be controlled by the influence of hypnosis. At the end of the day you'll also have a an understanding of how the mind of a person can be altered.

What Happens When You are Hypnotized

When you go into the state of hypnosis it is possible to describe the sensation as exactly like what you feel when daydreaming . You are able to imagine things you would normally not imagine, just like the way your mind works when you're in the state of dreaming when you sleep. Imagine flying, performing the real Superman punch and more; But the truth is, you're awake and focused.

What is the reason people believe that when you're being hypnotized, you're actually in a state of sleep? The reason is because when you're focused on something you wish to be aware of and you are distracted, you become lost. It's like watching a film as well as reading an article. you believe that any scenario could happen in real life and your thoughts are engrossed.

It is possible to suspend your belief for a short time and be open to the possibilities available to you. Much like reading books or watching a film, it is your choice to be convinced that the thing you are reading is actually happening in reality. It means you have the complete freedom to believe in or act during hypnosis. You are able to decide to defy the suggestion or an order that is made to you. If you do not choose to engage in hypnosis there's nothing an hypnotist can perform to force you to take something or to think of the thought.

What causes this? If you are able to access your subconscious during the midst of a hypnosis experience it can be that you feel like you're in a state of tranquility however, you're actually awake. Since you're allowing you to let go of thoughts and imaginations, the subconscious starts working behind the scenes and creates scenes and images in your mind. But, the conscious brain is active in your thoughts and you are able to recognize that certain things that you imagine could not be realized in reality. However, your subconscious might continue to permit you to take advantage of your feelings.

When your emotions are stimulated when your subconscious is able to project into your brain, you'll be able to form thoughts with your conscious mind. You may feel inspired or come up with a specific idea you are able to execute even though you're fully aware.

Like daydreaming, hypnosis may inspire you based on concepts that are in a story you read or were exposed to.

Following a hypnosis session you may feel the urge to do something you wouldn't even think about previously. In this case you're acting in response to the suggestions you have heard or seen however it's your decision to accept these suggestions. As you are extremely hypnotic and in a state, you might have a difficult time ignoring the idea, as if your brain is altered in a specific way.

Why Learn or Experience Hypnosis?

It is possible to be hypnotized by yourself. All you have to do is read an hypnosis hypnotic text or hear an audio track to put yourself in the state of trance. You can also utilize the suggestions you wish to modify.

The majority of people like the idea of being hypnotized or learning how to do it themselves , because of the following motives:

1. It allows them to do things that they usually don't allow themselves from doing.

Every person struggles with a particular way of living, and everyone would like to be in control of their behavior and beliefs particularly those which are hindering them from achieve their objectives. Certain people realize that their fears about themselves hinder them from achieving their talents.

Many people also struggle with negative habits they believe they can't remove from their daily routine. To be able to control routine behaviors, they'd have to accept the possibility that they're truly in charge.

2. It aids them to manage the pain and also reduce anxiety and stress.

The majority of the time, the phrase "mind is superior to matter" is the case. If your brain tells you that your back is like it was hit with the sledgehammer, your body will feel like that. This is the same when you're experiencing anxiety and stress - when you're compelled to believe that you are unable to handle the stress, your behavior will change to the thought. But, if you're capable of rewiring your mind to think differently and you'll be able to feel more relaxed.

3. It lets you trigger your confidence.

A few people think they're timid and intimidated by the people around them until they believe they can't be a good person even when others are watching. If this is the case for you, then make use of hypnosis in order to reveal your inner confidence.

4. It will help you figure out ways to become more efficient.

A few people are impeded by their daily routines to such an extent that they think it's impossible to come up with the most efficient and creative method of conducting business.

If they allow themselves to change the way they think about themselves, they are able to develop to more efficient ways of doing things that will help them achieve their goals quickly.

5. It helps you improve your communication and influence individuals.

Learn how to influence others with methods that you are able to apply in your everyday life will enable you to gain insight into the minds of other people. This can help you communicate concepts across and influence people, including those who appear to have a lot of obstacles to overcome. When you learn to better communicate and making the most of your suggestions you're creating opportunities that were impossible to reach previously.

These are just some of the things you can expect to enjoy when you master the art of hypnotizing and be attracted to. Nowis the time to master the fundamentals of this mind-bending method.

Chapter 2: The Playing with Suggestions

If you look at the way a suggestion box functions it will be apparent that it's a lot like to the way hypnotists work by manipulating the mind of an individual. The suggestion box is a repository of ideas about how an company should function and it's the responsibility of the company to apply these suggestions.

But, if nobody gets into the box, the ideas put there will never be noticed by the organization. If that is the case they will never get any clues regarding how others feel that their service could be better.

This is the same for your brain. If your mind was always in charge and in charge, you wouldn't be able open to any suggestions about what you could do to improve the way you act or think. If you go through hypnosis it is a conscious choice to let your mind rest in the background while letting your unconscious take over the steering wheel.

Your subconscious is the primary responsible for emotions and sensations which makes it vulnerable to hypnosis could let you experience feelings that you are trying to avoid and trigger emotions that let you experience your environment in a completely different way.

The Trick of the Mind using Suggestions

When you read "do not even think about the mug that holds your coffee" Your subconscious is doing reverse. At the time you saw it, you instantly thought of a mug that had coffee. It's the same when you are thinking of other negative words like "don't get caught late" and "don't be worried".

If those words say things you shouldn't do, your brain immediately imagines scenarios where you're late or you're stricken with anxiety. If these phrases are substituted with positive counterparts, such as "be punctual" or "find solutions to your issues" and your mind will create a scenario in your head where you're in a position to meet your deadlines and become a great troubleshooter. You can imagine these scenarios without having to enter the state of trance.

In this way it is possible to conclude that any hypnosis method won't work when you're unable to give the right suggestion to cause the image you would like to see in your mind. Keep in mind what your unconscious believes is the thing that it will create. It is the contents of your mind and the rest your body would shift to create the scene you thought of in your head.

Test Your Suggestion

Before you perform any hypnotic technique it is important to create a thought that is persuasive enough to spur a person to take an action. For instance, the idea you're looking to test is to make a pendant move in any direction you like in the event that you're holding it on the chain.

Then, test this for yourself. Imagine that you are superhuman and could move the pendant with just your brain. Through your mind's eye, watch the pendant move around in circles. Are you able to see that the necklace is moving? You can control it with your mind in the way that it'll go towards the reverse direction. Then, you can stop it.

What happened? The pendant didn't move simply because your mind instructed it to move - in actual fact, you are performing subtle movements using your fingers based on the idea that you're capable of using your brain to accomplish it.

If the pendant moves the pendant, you're essentially being hypnotized into believing that your mind is able to manipulate things telepathically. Now, you know that moving a thing by using your mind is a notion that people are able to act upon!

Making a Person Open Up to Suggestions

The act of hypnotizing someone has a drawback that not all people are willing to listen to suggestions, particularly when they don't like the person who is trying to seduce them. There are times when the person could appear as if they are having a hard in understanding what you're trying to communicate or is clearly resisting what you would like to say.

This is where the method of pacing and leading considered to be the most fundamental technique of hypnotism comes in handy. The term "pacing" means that you're transmitting an experience to your client, and then you are guiding him to the desired behavior that you would like to attain during your session of hypnosis.

What is the procedure? In this case, you would like to get your subject to scratch his hand. If you tell him what you would like him to perform There is an 80% chance that he'll do what you say. In fact, he might decide to avoid scratching any more.

Take note of what you'd think when you read this article:

While you are sitting there and regardless of the surroundings you're in, you're your attention is on the words you're reading right now and continue reading you are able to feel the sensation of tingling on the rear of your palm. Whatever you do, however you attempt to avoid it, you can't ignore the sensation that makes you'd like to scratch at the itch you feel in the middle, crawling and itching, on the side of your hand.

If you are in the midst of reading, sitting, and trying to not scratch you're getting the feedback about what's happening to you when you read the paragraph before. Since you are being told about what's happening to you in that moment, other feelings which may not be real begin to become part of your experience. The other sensation that wasn't there prior to that is the itching sensation, which is followed by the desire to scratch.

Hypnotic scripts are typically crafted in this way. To induce a person to feel or thinking about something that's not actually there You must tell him what you truly experience. The conscious mind will allow the statements because the subject is aware the reality of them is real. If you're confident that the person you are talking to is accepting feedback, it is the moment you encourage him to consider and feel another thing.

Leading and pacing requires timing. If you take your subject to lead until he becomes comfortable of the pace you are using, his mind will be able to snap back into the front seat instead of being in behind. This would instantly inform your subject that they are receiving false information. The subject will come back to a state of calm and behaving with confidence to being cautious. Do not worry too much , you can return to pacing so you please as long your participant remains engaged.

The Power of Confidence

If you're looking to become an effective hypnotist you must ensure that you're capable of effectively delivering a script for hypnosis. You might want to consider making a script before a mirror and recording your voice prior to attempting to trick people.

Why is this so important? It is because when you put someone in an hypnotic state in a hypnotic trance, you are essentially asking that they be attentive to you. Keep in mind that a person who is being hypnotized isn't at all relaxed or non-aware state. He is trying to concentrate on what you are saying and even a small change of your tone or indication that you're not certain of what you're doing could disrupt your concentration.

If your subject loses focus, he'll quickly think that he's being manipulated, or that you're not certain of the intention behind what you're trying accomplish. In this case the subject is unwilling to take part in any hypnotic activity you may attempt to perform the next time.

Can You Prevent Hypnosis?

If you don't wish to be hypnotized then there's nothing an hypnotist could perform to get you to enter the state of trance to induce hypnosis on you. Because you know the requirements to be hypnotized, are aware of the factors you should avoid doing to avoid being at risk of being hypnotized.

If you suspect the possibility that someone may be trying to seduce you by walking in a synchronized manner with your movements and trying to get in tune with you, the initial step you should do is change your movements without paying attention to the person you are hypnotizing. If you are not focused on his speed, there's no way that he will be able to get inside your head.

You can shift your attention to something else, and then think that you don't think you can trust the person trying to get in touch with you. If you can make these kinds of barriers that you can create, then you are protected from being affected.

Once you've mastered the fundamentals, it's time to master some tricks.

Chapter 3: How to Sell Anything

It's true that you can be attracted by the salesperson or view a commercial on TV. If you've ever felt like you're "hypnotized" to purchase the product you've seen on TV, you are probably.

How Do They Do That?

If you are watching an advertisement or feel pressured by a salesperson to purchase something you might not really require it is an entirely different type of pace. Psychologists refer to this kind of pacing future-pacing.

Future-pacing is when you inform your subject of what follows:

1. How will his future unfold?

It is possible that he will require a tool or any other product to resolve a problem that will likely to have to confront. For instance, if is the one to do the laundry himself and his washing machine failed it is most likely require the detergent that could enable him to clean his clothing.

2. How could he be unable to look for something he wants which could lead to him creating additional requirements that your product could meet to.

If he is aware that he will require detergent, it is possible to think of any detergent available on the market. However, this doesn't assure that it will meet all of his laundry requirements. This is when you are able to lead him to do the things you would like to see and that is to make him believe that he requires this laundry detergent that you're selling.

It is possible to suggest to him that if you find yourself in a situation where he has to wash his clothes so badly the job doesn't stop at ensuring the clothes are clean of staining. It must be odorless, germ-free and dry quickly. Since the washing machine broke down, he has to dry his laundry using air. Any brand he can think of doesn't provide an instant drying effect.

In this moment, he will be thinking that he would require a detergent that will let him dry his clothes quickly. Since everyone who is doing their laundry would need this feature, either regardless of whether they have the spin dryer it is an added benefit to the detergent you're selling. You've offered an offer to your customer and the subconscious of his will be thinking of his ideal future being capable of washing and drying his clothes without much effort.

3. Provide a product that can meet the future-pacing scenarios you've envisioned.

After you've created this scenario you would like to instil into his mind it is possible to demonstrate your product in a way that will solve the various scenarios that he's ever thought of , while keeping him on track for the future.

You could then create further scenarios to describe how thrilled he'll be when he is finally able to test the product you offer at home. It is possible to instill the future-pace idea by explaining the specifics of how the product is going to be utilized. The hypnosis process is complete.

If you think about it, the majority of ads don't need to wait long to perform this hypnotic trick. The only thing they need to do is catch your attention in the first few seconds and then provide the hook you'll be focused on. The second seconds following the hook will be the future-pacing scenario the brand would like to create.

Chapter 4: Setting up Your Hypnosis Session

Although it is possible to apply hypnosis to every day scenarios, that does not mean you'll be able to immediately influence everyone. Even if you're doing self-hypnosis, you'll still require setting up the proper environment to successfully hypnotize.

Remember to Break Down Barriers

Presupposition is an extremely effective method of hypnosis, specifically when you're dealing with a reluctant subject before you. For instance, if you have a child with an habit of staying up late and you're trying to get him to get to bed earlier however, you can't be certain that the child will respond to your suggestion. This is why it is best to cover your "orders" in your statement to express the information in a manner that it's more appropriate to the subject.

Instead of telling your child "You need to go to bed around 9pm" alternatively, use the phrase "You may choose to fall asleep approximately 8:30pm or 9pm since you've been a great boy today." Since you're capable of telling your child that they have the liberty to do whatever that he likes since he has the ability to behave in the manner you would want to, he will choose to take advantage of the two choices you've offered. Since he only has the thought of the hours between 8:30pm and 9pm and be aware that he could decide on the later time of going to bed, he will gladly go to bed when you would like him to.

Hypnosis and Leading

Presupposition is a technique for creating a future-pacing scenario that is perfect for creating the illusion that people had a similar experience before. One of the most effective examples is Kellog's Cornflakes commercial with the phrase "Have been able to forget how great the taste of these cornflakes?"

There is a chance that you don't enjoy cornflakes in any way or don't buy Kellog's products. However, this statement makes the impression that you used to like cornflakes in the past. Since it is targeted at your brain, you will feel vividly imagining the flavor of cornflakes even though it's not the truth.

That's why a majority of scripts of hypnotherapy contain lines that make use of presupposition. For instance, if would like to get your client to ease up, you could utilize phrases that read "You notice that your body feels relaxed and heavy." This would induce the subject to think of relaxation and believe that he's indeed relaxed.

Make Your Subject Focus Easier

If you wish to get your subject to be focused on your voice to ensure that he's taking note of your ideas, ensure that you speak with a calm and gentle voice. The reason for this is that People do not want to be captivated by any sound they don't want to hear. If your voice seems rough or uncertain, your listener would prefer to concentrate on a sound that they would find pleasant.

The majority of hypnotists wish to have their clients unwind in order to concentrate. If you've been watching the hypnosis session or are listening to audio hypnotherapy tracks, you will observe that they usually begin with a soothing sound track followed by an instruction to the person to shut his eyes. In this way they can provide a pleasant auditory experience, and remove the visual distraction. Once the listener is able to focus to the sound while keeping their eyes closed, the hypnosis process could begin.

Note: If it's impossible for your subject to keep his eyes shut as you try to seduce him in a setting in which he must remain aware, then you may prefer visual images to aid in removing distracting factors. A few use swinging pendulums or any other object that has the same rhythm that they want their subjects to fixate their attention on. It would be acceptable to not ask your subject to shut his eyes.

Induce and Deepen the Trance

Once your subject has become at ease and you know that he's able to keep his concentration, you can induce him to enter the state of hypnosis. In this phase you'll be capable of tapping into the subconscious of your subject and activate his senses by images.

As an example, you can make a guess that he feels his body is relaxed and, as long when his body is relaxed it is likely that he will think that in his mind that he's walking down a set of stairs. The top of the stairs is an entrance. When he opens it, you will be able to enter a gorgeous garden.

Through this visualisation by presenting this image, you're making him imagine a sequence of events. Because his brain has the power to decide what he will see He would surely like to know what's on the ground. It is likely that he's imagining what plants in your garden smell or how damp the grass is onto. The more details you give about the garden and the more you engage his senses in the

27

imaginary garden. In the end, all things happen within the subconscious mind, and that bring back memories of a real garden he was in.

Inducing trance with imagery, your aim is to let your subject be lost in the world of his imagination. The more imagery you use the more receptive the subject will be for your ideas.

Now you are able to tap into your unconscious to "obey" instructions for example, thinking that smoking cigarettes is unpleasant and that he might prefer to shed some weight, for instance, or any other thoughts you wish to embed in his mind. Once you've been able to establish these thoughts and he will have an idea of how to connect the behaviour you would like him to display with an action.

For instance, if you asked him to imagine an imaginary scene in which he's drinking coffee and reaching for cigarettes, and you created the impression that, in the imagined scene, he didn't like the taste of cigarettes and that experience then becomes permanent in his mind.

When he next thinks of having a smoke with the coffee, this experience might trigger and cause him to believe that smoking cigarettes isn't something he likes in any way.

But, be cautious - even though you may be thinking about things, his brain is always alert and ready to leap into the scene in the event that it believes something is wrong in the images.

Remember that people is only able to think of thoughts that they have encountered in the past. If the image you are talking about isn't clear the subject could be able to break out of the trance by using his own consciousness. For instance, if you try to get him to imagine a garden you have seen as a child and you say that you would come across a brook there and he is confused and leave the trance, if his memory states that there isn't a stream in the actual garden he been to at some point in time.

This is why you should ensure that you are creating images that are in his memory bank for that, you might need to know the subject's knowledge up to speed. If you're trying to attract a complete stranger, you might prefer to create images that will be familiar to him.

For instance, having the person imagine walking on a staircase before opening the door is a safe visualization because it's likely that the person has been through a door before and previously used stairs.

Chapter 5: What is Hypnotism

We're pleased to introduce the first section of the book. We'll be discussing X-Men here. It's true, it right. If you're familiar with any of Marvel's fantastic designs, you'd be aware about hypnotism.

The art of hypnotism involves manipulating minds. You've probably heard of the famous name Uri Gagarin who was one of the European that was among the very first person to demonstrate hypnotic abilities. He was also able to bend the shape of a spoon while on television. It's not true that we're going to learn on any magic tricks. What we will learn about is possible and is attainable, and by nobody else than you. Another definition of Hypnotism can be described as a state in which you are able to directly access your subconscious mind. This is truly remarkable. It's a state that demonstrates greater suggestion. When a suggestion is embraced by the intuition, it is then unquestionably monitored. It is a very common situation that people experience at least daily (cases are: the parkway being enthralling and wandering around in a fantasy world and so on).

The art of manipulating minds is known as the art of hypnotism. It's not just the power to cause minds to alter their thinking but also the ability to control the direction that change takes them to. When it comes to the topic of hypnosis, it refers to a state of consciousness that is mid-way from which a person's mind is the most likely to respond to suggestions and clues. In regards to what happens following the hypnosis experience, there are typically two theories.

The first theory, known as the modified theory, suggests that once you're placed in the state of hypnosis you are put into an euphoria state that is nothing more than your sleep consciousness. Also all remains the same apart from the activities of your brain and it's in a state of dormancy. The second theory suggests that once a person is hypnotized, they begin to behave as they imagine themselves, and not who they really are. The second theory affirms that a state called being hypnotized is simply a the state of playing a role.

To try is to Perfect.

The practice of hypnotizing makes one perfect. In the same way, effective hypnotizing is necessary to become an excellent performer. As they say that to make the future in a neat manner it is important to have studied the past with care. Now, we are reading the past.

To enjoy the hypnotic sensation it is necessary to be able to see the term from a professional standpoint instead of a dilettante's perspective in which a person is seduced into a deep sleep in which the subconscious part of him awake than before before, eliminating the external distractions. Professionals don't glance at flowers. We look at the root. In the same way, we attempt to comprehend the concept of hypnosis as described through the pioneers.

As we delve into the history to find James Braid, a Scottish surgeon, as one of the pioneers of Hypnosis and also the first to create the term. Braid initially stated that Hypnosis is a form of sleep that was a nervous one that was distinct from the usual one, and described it as "A particular condition that affects the nervous system, caused by a deliberate and abstracted concentration of the visual and mental eye on a single thing, and that is not arousing experience" And then continued to redefine the term "hypnosis" as a state of mind incineration which often results in an enlightened state of relaxation, which he coined "nervous sleeping". As time passed, the doctor admitted the fact that his terminology was erroneous and inaccurate. He was however adamant at the notion that "Nervous sleep" could be a better alternative to the term monoideism, which referred to the splintering group of subjects with amnesia-like symptoms.

Michael Nash provides a list of eight definitions for the term "hypnosis" by various authors, as well as his personal belief that the practice of hypnosis is "a particular instance in psychological regression"

Janet at the beginning of the century and later, Ernest Hilgard has described hypnosis as a process of dissociation.

Psychologists from the social sciences Sarbin as well as Coe have studied hypnosis in terms of the theory of roles. Hypnosis plays a role individuals play, and they behave "as as" they were being hypnotized.

T. X. Barber identified hypnosis in terms nonhypnotic behavioral characteristics like motivation for tasks and the act of identifying the state of mind as hypnosis.

When he wrote his first works, Weitzenhoffer defined that hypnosis is a state that is more suggestible. Recently, he has described hypnotism as "a kind of influence that an individual exerted upon an individual through the agent or medium or suggestion."

Psychoanalysts Gill and Brenman explained hypnosis using the psychoanalytic idea of "regression for the benefit of the self."

Edmonston has characterized the hypnosis phenomenon as just a relaxation state.

Spiegel And Spiegel have suggested that hypnosis has a biological capacity.

Erickson is regarded as the most prominent advocate of the idea that hypnosis is a specific internal-directed, altered state of being.

Joe Griffin and Ivan Tyrrell (the creators of the human givens method) define the term "hypnosis" as "any artificial method of accessing an REM state, which is the state of the brain where dreams take place" and claim that this definition, when understood correctly, can solve "many of the mysteries , and debates concerning the subject of hypnosis". [23]

As the years passed, in 2005, it was through the Society for Psychological Hypnosis, Division 30 of the American Psychological

Association the formal definition was given. "Hypnosis usually includes an introduction to the method where the person is told that suggestions for experiences of imagination will be offered. The hypnotic introduction (this is the procedure of placing a person in an hypnotic state) is an extended first suggestion to use the individual's imagination. It could also be further elaborated upon from the introduction. What is meant to stimulate and push the subject to assess their the response to suggestions is is known as the hypnotic process. If hypnosis is used, one individual (referred to as"the subject) is directed by another (referred by the term hypnotist) to react to suggestions for changes to the subjective experience, changes in perceptions, sensations, emotions or thoughts".

The report also included the following remarks with regard to the fact that hypnosis is a form of hypnosis "Hypnosis usually begins with an intro to the process in which the person being hypnotized is informed that suggestions for imagining experiences will be given. The hypnotic introduction is an extended suggestion to engaging one's imagination. It could include further explanations of the introduction. A hypnotic technique is employed to encourage and measure reactions to suggestions. Through hypnosis, one individual (the person who is the subject) is assisted by another (the person who is hypnotized) to make suggestions that suggest changes to perception, changes of perception, feeling, or thought. People can also learn self-hypnosis that is the process of executing hypnotic techniques by themselves. If the subject reacts to hypnotic prompts then it is usually assumed that hypnosis is caused. Many believe that hypnotic reactions and experiences are typical of a state of hypnosis. Some believe it's not necessary utilize the term "hypnosis" in connection with the induction process, some believe it is essential"

A look at technicalities

As the first step in becoming a professional, we break in to the myths and the facts:

The myth that some people aren't able to be attracted to.

The truth is that although some scientists and doctors assert that certain people cannot be hypnotized, all people have the capacity to be hypnotized as it's a normal, natural state that we goes through at least two times per every day - when we wake up and going to sleep. It is also possible to go into a state of hypnosis whenever we are completely absorbed in a television or film show. If the actors are their characters within our heads, we become completely absorbed. Additionally, if we're driving and daydreaming to the point that we skip a turn or freeway exit that we are familiar with the exit, it is likely that we were in an euphoric state.

Many people have this belief because of a negative experience they've experienced with an magician. People respond to different strategies, and even in the event that a particular method isn't working previously, then it's just a decision to find the approach that is most effective for them. IMDHA Certified Hypnotherapists/Hypnotists have several techniques that they can use, and are trained to find a method that will work best for you.

Myth that you can be manipulated to perform actions against your own will

In reality, the hypnosis expert is just a guide, or facilitator. He/she is not able to "make" you to do anything that is against your wishes. In reality when you are in a hypnotic state you're fully aware of the entire situation. If you don't like the way the hypnotist has you, you are given the ability to refuse the advice.

It's a common notion that is rooted in stage plays and other events that make use of this "power" that is the magician. It's important to note that sometimes an identical issue is discussed in the form of "Can people be hypnotized to do things that they would never usually be able to do?" Of course, the answer can be "Yes" once you consider that the goal of hypnosis is usually to change the way we do things that we've been doing before. It is important to note that these changes aren't at the discretion of the client. Hilgard's (1977) research at Stanford revealed a concept called "The Secret Observer" which suggests that there's a component of the client that monitors the hypnotic process , and can prevent them from responding in a manner that does not conform to their moral and ethical norms.

Myth: When you are hypnotized, you'll always speak the truth and may even reveal secrets about your personal life

The truth is that you can lie under hypnosis the same way as you would in waking. Since the hypnosis state gives you access to your unconscious and resources, you might be in a position to create more inventive illusions while in a trance. Furthermore, you're in total control of what you decide to reveal or hide.

Myth: I'll forget what the hypnotist has said.

In reality, everyone experiences hypnosis in a different way ... depending on the person. For certain people it's a state of mind in which you're at the forefront of the hypnotist's words and paying more attention and for others, it's more of a being in a state of mind where your attention could shift between thoughts ... often without paying focus on the words of the hypnotist. Any way you choose to go is fine and neither is more or less effective than the others. It's just a matter of your individual style.

Myth: One could be stuck in a trance for the rest of their lives.

The truth is that no one has ever been caught in a hypnotic state. Hypnosis is an naturally occurring state in which can be entered and left in the course of an entire day. There are no reported or reported risks in hypnosis when working with a qualified practitioner. If the hypnotist does not manage to free the person from hypnosis then they returns to a fully alert state by themselves. In response to the individual's need to sleep, they will orally drift to sleep, or simply regain consciousness in a matter of minutes.

While in the state sleep, our brainwaves fluctuate across those Alpha and Theta ranges. When you decide to let go of the hypnosis no matter what the reason, it is possible to get your eyes open and be fully awake. If you were doing self-hypnosis prior to sleeping and ended up in that Delta state, it could mean that you'd go to sleep.

The myth that intelligent people aren't able to be controlled by hypnosis

The truth is that, contrary to popular belief research suggests that those with above average ability to concentrate, being focused and possess an ability to think creatively and a vivid imagination typically are the most successful subjects.

Myth: Someone who is under the influence of hypnosis sleeps or is unconscious.

The truth is that hypnosis does not imply consciousness or sleep however a popular belief is that you're asleep while hypnotized. The feeling of a formal inducing hypnotic state could be similar to sleep from a physical perspective like slowed breathing eyelids closed muscles relaxed, and activities reduced. From a mental perspective, the person is usually relaxed and awake, in a relaxed state that allows the individual to think or talk, and move around if required. All clients are different and experience hypnosis in the way that is unique to them. Some people are so comfortable with the procedure that they find themselves drifting into and out of a dream-like state. In certain instances, they may respond without thinking, via an ideomotor signal or some other method. Although it is not widely used however, there are some instances where under the supervision by a specially trained hypnotherapist may induce unconsciousness for reasons of surgical anesthesia or the treatment of acute pain or in situations of emergency that warrant it.

The Myth that Hypnosis may be in contradiction to religion

The fact is that hypnosis is a method to reduce or alleviate pain, to overcome anxieties, fears as well as addiction issues and others. While some religious groups have expressed reservations to hypnosis, all religious communities are in agreement with the application of hypnosis to help people. This includes Roman Catholic, Orthodox, and the majority of Protestant Christian Churches as well as Judaism, Hinduism, Buddhism and many more. Hypnosis does not belong to any of the major religions of the world. An ethical and professional hypnotist is respectful of the beliefs of his clients and does not employ it to alter an individual's beliefs about religion.

The next step in becoming a professional, or the layman, is knowing the concept of hypnotism to which we need first grasp the technical terms used and the explanations of the defined definitions.

Suggestion:

A person with no sense of light or to shed could believe these suggestions to be words used by the hypnotist in order to make the person to relax and focus. However, as hypnotists, we have to know more. The better part is this. Like all fields this one has its own set of conflicting ideologies. How the term'suggestion is interpreted by the hypnotists is an example of that is a source of conflict. A particular hypnotist's ideological stream considers they are a method for communicating between the person who is hypnotized as well as the conscious mind and on the other end of the spectrum there are hypnotists who insist that the word refers to the appeal of the person who is hypnotized to the subconscious or, if not coined the unconscious portion of mind. Sigmund Freud as well as Pierre Janet brought these concepts to light during the late 19th century. Sigmund Freud created a theory known as the Psychoanalytic Theory, which explains the concept the consciousness line thoughts are set up on the brain's surface and the unconscious lines are hidden beneath the mind's surface.

Subject:

The subject is the person who is being controlled by the person who is hypnotizing them. These are people who have turned to hypnosis for an option to get through issues, or overcome their worst fears or anxieties that have kept them from their lives. This may not be as simple, but can be broader, physical illnesses can be treated by using hypnosis.

Hypnotist:

Here we are. We are here! We're not the only ones! It's not even a possibility. This is what we are, after intense training and deep understanding about the techniques used in the art of hypnosis. In general an hypnotist is an individual who, has completed years of practice and theoretical education is prepared enough to guide the client to hypnosis and obtain the results the person wants to achieve.

It is important to come to the realization that the hypnotist and the subject should not always be two distinct people. That is there's no requirement for two people to is hypnotized. The hypnotist could also be the person who is subject to hypnosis, and in that case, self-hypnosis is also referred to as self-hypnosis. Self-hypnosis refers to the practice of giving hypnotic exercises to self. Self-hypnosis is a method to gain self-control. It can be employed to control your thoughts cravings, desires, and urges. Apart from the reasons mentioned above in the previous paragraph, it can also be utilized to manage your mental state overall. Let's start the journey with no further delay.

Minds that are conscious and subconscious

When we discover that hypnosis is involves the subconscious aspect of this subject matter, we may be able to clarify what is the subconscious mind. Imagine the subconscious mind as a place where you store everything that's not in your conscious brain.

The conscious mind (10-12 %) The Conscious Mind (10-12 %): In normal circumstances, you're only conscious of the thoughts that are happening within your mind. You are able to think about the challenges which are right in front of your face and, as you speak, and consciously attempt to recall where you put your keys. While doing all this your conscious mind works closely with your subconscious mind.

It's similar to the CPU in an electronic computer that is operating under the current laws of the game.

Its tasks include thinking, locating the logic, feeling and making decisions, analyzing, and controlling body movement

The conscious mind works out will power, which is what we refer to as.

It's also the site that stores working memory (memory we use on a daily basis to perform).

Subconscious mind:

The subconscious mind is able to store every single one of your life experiences and beliefs, as well as your memories, your skills and all the situations you've gone through and all the images you've ever witnessed.

The best method to grasp the mind of your subconscious is to consider the scenario of a person who would like to learn to drive the car. At first, he would not be able to have conversations with others when driving, because the mind is focused on the different movements that are involved. It's because he's still operating his brain to drive.

Your subconscious mind, your Autopilot!

A few weeks later, driving becomes the norm and happens in a way that is not requiring anyone thinking about it. The driver could also begin using his mobile phone or calling his companions while driving.

The driving habits have been transfered to the subconscious, and consequently, his conscious mind became free. This enabled him to to talk on his cellphone.

The mind of the subconscious the one responsible for the automatic triggers of emotions and feelings occur when you are confronted with the new environment. If you are planning to present a talk, then the fear and anxiety that you could be experiencing are actually created as a result of your mind's subconscious.

The conscious mind in turn the one responsible for logical thinking, calculation and all actions executed while you're conscious. Your subconscious also manages the other bodily functions like heartbeats, breathing, and breathing.

Another example that could help you understand your subconscious is the breathing process. Before you began reading the previous paragraph, your breath was controlled by the subconscious.

Now, I would like you to take a moment to manage your breathing for a minute. It will be possible to do that, naturally. The first time, it was the conscious mind that was directing your breathing. However, when you lose your attention, the subconscious will take over.

Program your subconscious mind

If the information regarding driving is stored in your subconscious mind , it is stored as an program. Consider your brain as an electronic computer, and the information about driving is a program that can executed automatically when needed.

It's the same for a lot of other actions and emotions. If someone has offended you, the program that you have installed to repress anger is likely to begin and the outcome is a behavior you will regret in the future.

Through programming your subconscious mind with new programming, you will be able to solve many issues in your life. Make sure that your autopilot is able to run the system without disrupting your life or causing any issues.

The process of programming your subconscious mind can be achieved via the use of hypnosis. Your subconscious brain learns through repetition, not by logic. This is why you are able to convince that someone to believe an idea by repeating the same argument over and over again, rather than using logic. For more details on this subject, check out our guide for the science behind convincing

The rules of the subconscious mind

In order to maximize the potential of your subconscious mind, you need to first understand how your subconscious mind functions. It is guided by a variety of rules.

Understanding these guidelines will allow you to make the most effective use that part of the mind, with the most effort. In the end of this page is a hyperlink that provides all the information you require to learn about the rules of the subconscious mind.

Ego defense mechanisms

Like your body has developed defenses against physical traumas and injuries, your subconscious mind also has its defenses against emotional trauma and wounds.

These are called ego defense mechanisms or unconscious defense mechanisms. The mechanism's primary role is to guard your wellbeing and assist you in overcoming emotional shocks.

The subconscious mind and forgetting about someone else

The reason that people remain broken after breaking up is because they hold false notions about relationships that are stored in their minds. My book How to conquer anyone in a matter of days, I explained how removing notions such as "the the one" as well as "the soul the one" make to forget about anyone in a the space of a few days.

Once someone is rid of these notions, they will see that he will eventually meet a person who will replace the person who left and thus recovery takes place.

By bringing your subconscious and your conscious mind

The subconscious and the conscious mind could make a fantastic team when you use them together. The first one can take care of some tasks and then delegate them to the second , while the second sends messages and feedback about the job through emotions towards the primary.

The emotions are nothing more than messages that your subconscious mind to inform you of something. When you learn how to make the most efficient use of the co-operation between your subconscious and conscious mind, your abilities will grow and you will enjoy more control over your emotions.

How can hypnosis affect the your subconscious mind?

Hypnosis is a method of providing the subconscious or unconscious mind with fresh and beneficial information, like changing the programming of computers.

Hypnosis can be a great method to bypass this critical filter. In hypnosis, the crucial filter shuts down for a period of time. The conscious mind remains awakeand is able to make choices. But you're now in control as your subconscious is open to any suggestion your conscious mind would like to accept.

Induction:

A situation in which the person, (The person who is being is being hypnotized) responds to messages, suggestions or communication made by the person who is hypnotized (The person who is hypnotized) is known as Hypnotic Induction. We will also learn the meaning of Induction and the techniques used to achieve it.

What is the reason for the inducement? The hypnotist, in order to uncover or to rekindle old memories, sends subjects into a hypnotic state of trance. The purpose of the induction could be to simply open the blockages and bring back memories or to discover specific information, which is blurred in the depths of the unknown. It could also mean to do nothing at all and nothing else than to let go.

How can I incite?

The second major question. There are a variety of ways that a magician can influence the subject. The essentials, rules you be required to understand prior to beginning to learn about hypnosis techniques is

1. Find an area of interest

Choose a subject that must be willing to serve as the guinea pig for your hypnosis test. The person you choose to use for your experiment must be aware of all the things you will conduct to him in full. In obtaining the consent from the person you are talking to is of paramount importance due to ethical considerations. It is important to inform them all the information you'll be saying in order to build their confidence. The purpose of hypnotizing someone is more getting their trust than making them to fall asleep. If the person you are hypnotizing is confident that they're in good in their hands, then the majority of your job is done right there and then.

2. Ask about previous experiences

Engage in a conversation with your subject about previous experiences, or encounters with hypnotism anytime or anywhere during their life. Talk to them about the experience and the way they responded to it. This will assist you in determining the type of issue you're working with.

3. Reassurance

It is vital that your subject be capable of trusting your guidance as a guide. Make sure that your subject is assured that they'll recall every single detail they were asked about or said during the conversation following using hypnosis. I'll reveal the truth here: this is a fake. They won't recall everything they said, however telling them this increases confidence.

4. Place

Pick a cozy area to do the hypnosis. The location should be lit and peaceful. You should ensure that no disturbances can penetrate the area during the duration of time you'll be working.

5. To stimulate an idea

Begin by asking the subject to shut their eyes and go to the blissful world that they have created. Then, imagination is a factor because it is all about the extent to which the subject can think. You can come up with your own ideas, like a lush green meadow with a clear, crystal-clear stream that flows through.

6. Complete the form with all the information.

Once you've created an idea in your subject's head and helped them move towards what they believe is their ideal place to be now is the now time for them to fill up their brains with little but intricate details. Find out what they notice surrounding them when they're strolling in their blissful place. You can ask them about what color their shoes are or the form the top of their dress. These aren't details, however, as you ask the subject is constantly creating. Therefore, you're not asking the right questions to create, but rather helping create.

7. Instruct

Change your tone from a suggestion to instructive. Make use of phrases like "Do it" instead of asking ''would you like to try it gradually but surely, the person will fall into your manipulative trap and begin repeating your message or responding to the questions you say. Don't cross the ethical boundaries of not asking any questions that they wouldn't want to respond to in normal situations.

8. Provide Positivity

While the person is in a state of hypnosis affirmations which are encouraging and positive in the nature. If your session is to help the subject to let go of a habit that is harmful speak to them in an encouraging tone and using positive words such as:

"You are entitled to be better than falling victim to this habit"

"I believe in you. You can overcome this"

"There is nothing you can't do."

Don't give up; be persistent and it will get better."

9. A Slow End

The most effective way to conclude this hypnosis exercise is to say loudly, stating that you're going to count to five at the time of which they'll slowly awake from their sleep. With a firm tone begin counting from one to five and with the minimum of two seconds space between consecutive number.

10. Relax

Do not engage your person in intense and exhausting activities right after they've woken. Allow them to be alone, and tell them not to dwell about what occurred. Inform them that they've done a fantastic job and are now free of any issues they may have had.

Depth Levels of Hypnosis:

Certain people will experience more intense level of relaxation than other. The deeper levels, the greater the degree of influence your suggestions will have. As a stage-subliminal specialist It is essential to understand the various profundity degrees that are involved in Hypnosis and the related manifestations of each. There are four key phases of Hypnosis:

1) Hypnotical;

2) Light Trance;

3) Medium Trance; and

4.) Deep Trance, also known as "Sleepwalking," a state that allows an individual to perform actions that are appropriate to the wake state, but is actually deeply asleep. People who talk or walk while asleep are exhibiting somnambulistic behaviour.

Key Factor of Deep Hypnosis:

The reality of the situation is that everyone are hypnotized to a certain extent, on the other hand it is rated about 20% of people are somnambulists. They are also referred by the term "hypnotics"-people who are able to go into deep hypnosis. This tiny, yet appealing segment of the population are the ideal performers for an enthralling stage show. It's not to suggest that every subject who is not somnambulists should be excluded from your training. In fact, the contrary is true. If you can figure out how to successfully hypnotize people with less sleep-inducing capabilities, you'll be more skilled in handling highly attractive subjects before an audience.

Alongside the normal capacities that you can use, there are two aspects that impact a person's ability to be in a state of hypnosis-cooperation (either conscious or not) and the ability to inspire. This new variable is typically amplified in an inner-charged event, like performing live. The magnificent lighting as well as the music, crowd, and desire of rare occasions on an arena are all geared to boost the impact.

Another point to note is that the ability of a person to enter hypnotic states will increase through each successful hypnosis experience. This is the basis that underlies the "rehypnotization" method. It's a formidable tool to rapidly extend hypnosis to extremely hypnotic subjects and also sorting out those who aren't.

Rehypnozization

Rehashed hypnotization's makes it easier for a person to be able to enter Hypnosis. It's like competing athletes preparing their bodies for a specific manner, but the subject who is hypnotized is shaping his or her own psyche. Every time a person experiences the hypnosis, and then stirs the ability of that person to pay attention more intensely and focus on the advice of the administrator is improved.

This concept is the basis of hypnotization, which implies that you must have to be honest to be able to understand. It's an extent a successful tool to improve the quality of hypnosis even in the most powerless individuals, particularly after a rapid (mass) stimulation to an audience. Additionally it provides an unbeatable tool for screening those who do not have the capability to engage in deep hypnosis.

This is how it will meet your expectations. The group of people who will be taking part in the this stage is told that in one minute, you'll wake them all at once. As they get their eyes open the simple strategies listed below can help that you achieve the highest possible levels of hypnosis for your subject and in the process, you will achieve the greatest degree of sensitivity to your ideas. If they close their eyes and look at yours, they'll go back into a more deep, more steady sleep than at any time in recent. The administrator gets to each subject and asks them to examine his eyes. He advises "Your eyes are becoming heavier, extremely heavy. They can't be open anymore, so close your eyes and take a nap. If anyone fails to respond and then re-enter hypnosis again, that individual is immediately disqualified. After that, the remaining conscious subjects are woken in a group and informed when they look into the eyes of the specialist who is hypnotizing them and fall further into a much more restful sleep. The subjects who are unable to focus are disqualified. The subjects could now be offered a group test along with a (compound) suggestion that the test's completion will bring them to a lower level. It's a thought. This method works, so use it.

More Strategies

Alongside the most effective timing, reiteration, and the presentation of ideas There are many methods to gain an advantage in the field of influencing the subject:

1. Create early wins. Because the impact of your advice grows with each achievement, and diminishes with each failure, always begin with tests that give you the greatest chance of success, and then progress gradually more difficult ones.

2. Insist on establishing a pattern of conformity. Involuntary responses to commands improve the acceptance of involuntary suggestions later. Also, when you ask a subject to stand or sit or stretch his arm in a particular manner and so on. In the absence of any criticism, the way that the subject follows can often translate into suggestions to hypnotize.

3. Check to increase the effectiveness of a recommendation. Any time you feel it's appropriate you are able to recommend it

upon the basis that is three or five and so on. The subject is likely to do as. This intense system assists in identifying the subject precisely as the exact moment in which a craving response is typical.

4. Make use of non-verbal ideas to strengthen verbal ones. Dramatic artistry is an essential aspect of stage and hypnosis. Non-verbal suggestions as physical signs, body changes as well as breathing, influence the outcome.

5. Utilize the power of mass proposals. The recommendations to a group like the board of trustees tend to be more effective than recommendations for a single subject. Participants in a group are more likely to overcome their barriers and are affected by the positive reactions of various members of the group.

Working with individuals:

The first step to mastering the art of hypnotism is to figure out how to activate hypnosis the individual subject. This is among the most crucial abilities you can acquire and its dominance is crucial to further development as a specialist in hypnosis. The most effective method of enforcing Hypnosis is usually initiated by acknowledgment. The person making the acknowledgement either intentionally or without knowing. In any scenario, the end result is the same: the person "expects" to become attracted to a hypnotic state. It is essential to understand that there are countless methods of hypnosis in the presence of. There isn't a that is a right or wrong approach. They all work in that they give assurance to the administrator as well as confidence to the person who is using it, as discussed the first chapter. The principal reason for any technique for hypnosis is that it allows the subject to focus the attention of the subject and to eliminate most of the unpleasant effects while still leaving only one source of advice that is usually that of the hypnosis expert as well as the ear of the person who is hypnotized.

The so-called passes-the use arms and hands to direct energy towards the subject in the process of induction are completely unnecessary. They are a remnant from the 18th century. In fact, even in this fashion, many modern performers still use the same emotional signals to demonstrate an acting technique. It's fine, in the sense that it is understood there is no scientific basis for their use. Also, there is no reason to make contact with a person's brow or knees, etc.-in general, no significant contact is required. The voice of a person is a good way to communicate.

Try the hypnotic affectation technique, one-on one, with many subjects until you've developed the capacity to influence the majority of them. Each outside distraction needs to be eliminated or reduced to the minimum feasible. From the beginning, be prepared to allow for a minimum of 10 minutes or more an individual to reach the state of hypnosis. Be careful not to over-exaggerate that rate is a factor in the duration. The most important thing to consider when starting out is to take in the most efficient system possible.

One of the main components of the most popular hypnotic stimulation techniques is the focusing of the subject's attention to an "object of fascination." The object is then kept or suspended about one foot in front of the subject. It must also be placed at a level that is just right (over the head of the subject) that it prompts the person to lift the eyes slightly towards the sky to consider thoughts. This is a good position for eye strain, which can unintentionally, have the same position as regular sleeping.

If you're wondering about what you could have to get to focus on, it could be a gemstone, coin ball, emblem, or even a pocket watch hanging from a chain. These are often connected to a sleep-inducing actuation system in popular media. objects that reflect light back towards the subject are the best for this purpose.

Chapter 6: The Case for Hypnotism

It is rare to see hypnosis used in the manner that the media and pop culture specifically depicts it. There's no clever taskmaster that flies around with an electronic watch in a pocket or who's eyes whirl fast before your eyes to make you feel swayed or perhaps intriguing. Also, it's not about how the character of Rosario Dawson in the film Trance transforms James McAvoy's character to Thomas Crown, how the stunning looks of the famed Hypno Toad are adored or amazing promises of wealth and happiness, as well as sexy bodies made by Paul McKenna.

There are still ongoing debates, discussions or disagreements continue to rage about the possibility that hypnosis is a viable option apart of making a normal person behave like an animal at the touch of a hypnotist's finger which is assuming that it's actually feasible of course. There are also discussions on self-hypnosis. One thing everyone can accept is that the practice of hypnosis doesn't work suitable for all. It's sometimes difficult for you to demonstrate that it can have an effect on certain people since its effects or credibility can't be verified in a way that is objective, i.e., with figures and statistical analysis. For things like manufacturing or pharmaceuticals it is possible to measure the outcomes using numbers and conduct statistical analysis on the results. In hypnosis, the only thing that you can rely on is the words spoken by those who were at the time of being hypnotized.

Therefore, the issue is more pressing is: can hypnosis actually work or is it actually true? Is it possible to conclude that the United States Military made the error of investing a lot of hours and dollars on hypnosis in order to enlighten the masses or is it true that hypnosis exists since the military actually used it? Do we have the ability to be certain that famous hypnotists such Keith Barry and Paul McKenna are simple people who are hucksters?

My belief that hypnosis can be a valid method of achieving results is clearly demonstrated through the writing of this book. Let me present an argument for the use of hypnosis using these evidences that I believe convincing enough to merit your more research on the subject.

Hypnosis and Kicking The (Smoking) Habit

It appears that famous hypnotists such as Paul McKenna aren't as hucksters like the anti-hypnosis crowd claim they are. McKenna has earned a lot of money from selling his self-help items which include audiobooks, books as well as videos and seminars. In all of them his books, he promises of earning money as well as losing weight and quitting smoking cigarettes.

At the very least, he's right when it comes to getting rid of smoking. What can I say? It is true that there are numerous published studies which have proven the use of hypnosis to be extremely efficient in helping smokers stop smoking. What is the exact effectiveness?

Think about the fact that on average it was discovered that hypnosis had an 90.6 percent chance of getting rid of the habit in six months to three years. It was also found that 87% of those who had hypnotherapy to quit reported that they continued to stay away from the nicotine temptations after more than three years. So, the question is why do nicotine patches continue selling like hotcakes?

Hypnosis Has Been Used as A Substitute for Drugs

It's been proven that hypnosis may help satisfy cravings for lower-level substances like cigarettes, can it work with more potent substances such as meth, cocaine, and other illicit drugs? Studies have found that hypnosis can significantly enhance the likelihood of getting rid of dependence to these powerful drugs and remaining completely clean. The study that was conducted during - - when else? the 1960s, tried to determine whether those mind altering "benefits" from LSD could be replicated with the substance. The results? It is indeed possible to get it accomplished. This study managed achieve this simply by asking participants to reflect on what they experienced as well as how they were feeling that last occasion when they took LSD.

Then why do people want to use such substances in their bodies if the sole reason, i.e., the "high" is quickly acclimatized to the help of hypnosis? It is only logical sense since hypnosis is all about stimulating the subconscious mind, which is exactly what hallucinogenic substances like LSD actually accomplish.

A lot of creative geniuses have been known to utilize medications for "unleash" their creativity through tapping into their unconscious minds. Consider the surrealist writer Andre Breton. He relied on occasional hypnosis in order to encourage himself to write more naturally.

Cure for The Head and Missing Limbs

Maybe the word "cure" may not be the best word to employ. However, hypnosis - which is focused on tapping into your unconscious mind is an effective method to deal with mental health issues or issues. Numerous studies have proven that hypnosis - which puts people into the state of trance, and advising them that they're not or aren't as anxious or depressed - can have positive effects on managing emotional or mental issues. Hypnosis can be utilized to decrease or diminish anxiety around surgeries, both in the prior and post-surgery phases especially for those who aren't willing to undergo the procedure due to fear or a belief that isn't true.

Hypnosis has also been proven by research to be a reliable treatment for what's known as Phantom Limb Syndrome, which is the condition where people who have lost limbs still feel like it's there. The issue is in the feeling of "intense discomfort" in limbs which have gone away. Hypnosis may help lessen, diminish or even treat Phantom Limb Syndrome.

It's All About the Glaze

We're not talking about chicken, donuts or any other tasty food items. We're talking about eyes for subjects of hypnosis. Again there's no talk of covering the eyes with caramel.

Okay, now that I've got removed that issue and we can get back to hypnosis, and glaze do we? One of the strongest arguments against hypnosis and particularly stage hypnosis is that it requires all the parties involved to be fully aware of the process in order to be effective. In simple terms, it is believed that the person who is supposed to be hypnotized must "fake" to appear as if they are. However, science has come to help!

Researchers from three renowned European universities which include the University of Skovde (Sweden), University of Turku (Sweden) and Aalto University (Finland) - have studied the effects of hypnosis on the subjects eye. They mainly studied the ability of a woman to go into a state of hypnotic relaxation very fast, almost in an instant after speaking a word.

While she was in the hypnotic trance and was in a hypnotic trance, the team used several technological devices to monitor any changes to her eyes before and after the hypnotic Trance. They also discovered that, under the conditions of a true hypnotic trance eyelids of the person were blurred. While I'm not sure about the rest of you, but eyes that are glazed can be extremely difficult to recreate, in the absence of an alien or something.

The fact that subjects under hypnosis eyelids become dry is another convincing argument for the convincing case for the practice of hypnosis.

Memory Boost

For many self-help experts, one of their most well-known but often unfulfilled or misused -

promises is significant improvements in memory. They even go even further, saying that they will help you become better at public speaking as well as ensure that you won't lose your car keys, also prevent the countless other issues which are impacted by weak memory.

Although the most popular or popular method to improve memory is through mental organization of the memories of e.g. memory filing cabinets or storage cabinets, hypnosis is an alternative that is much more simple and more effective - method to increase memory. Although there is a lot of debate regarding whether it can actually help to remember more things however, studies do suggest that it could. Since both hypnosis and improved memory are all about accessing the part of the brain that's typically difficult or even impossible to access at a conscious level it makes sense to use hypnosis in the context of improving memory.

Sleight of Mouth Exists

It's a fact that the principle behind almost all tricks magicians employ is sleight of hands and is about hand movements used to hide or reveal what must be revealed in order to make the appearance of magic. Although magic doesn't exist however, sleight-of-hand is real. It's the reason magic appears real.

Although hypnosis isn't magical in that the magic trick is simple tricks, they both rely on sleight tactics. The distinction the fact that magical tricks depend on sleight-of-hand, while the hypnosis method relies on sleight of hand. It's part of an activity known as covert hypnosis which is the exact opposite of used in stage hypnosis. The difference with covert hypnosis, is that it is not like the stage or complicit hypnosis that is able to make people aware that they are being hypnotized, it is where subjects are hypnotized without their awareness. Scary!

It's not. It's basically the same as the use of subliminal images to hypnotize subjects - as in every commercial and advertisement is trying to communicate to unaware consumers. This is where activated or trigger words or phrases are repeatedly spoken to the subject while they're in a highly suggestive mental state. The subconscious hypnosis process suggests to subjects' minds that they are not being observed. It's similar to what Joseph's character and Leo do in the film Inception but it occurs while the subject is awake.

Famous People Use It

It's true that it's quite superficial and a shallow argument against hypnosis but when famous people have used it and are successful this means that hypnosis is real and works. Think of one of the top golfers of all time since the beginning of time - Tiger Woods. He utilized hypnosis as method of blocking out all distractions so that he could focus fully on his game. It's true that almost everything is absent, except mistresses. Yet, you cannot dispute his incredible golfing achievements and hypnosis has was a big help.

Albert Einstein was also known to use hypnosis, especially self-hypnosis. And legend claims that it was during the trance of one of him that he capable of formulating theories of relativity. If there's no cool benefit of hypnosis, then I do not know what is!

The Government Uses It

The U.S. Government, particularly through the CIA has conducted and continues to carry out obscure and even secret activities such as for instance the MKUltra Mind Control program. The program was born out of hypnosis studies conducted by the government and as part of the scheme, American war veterans and young men were all subjected to torture and drugs in the interest of studying the mind's control. Although the program has evolved from its beginnings however, its origins can be traced back to the hypnosis process, which indicates that the government recognizes its core. In some documents classified several many years back, evidence of the efficacy of hypnosis when interrogating people was stated through the CIA. These studies show that the effectiveness of hypnosis was greater in those who were asleep and doing their best to not get into a trance state and also when their personality was already intriguing.

Long History of Being Studied

A large portion of the evidence gathered by the CIA in support of the use of hypnosis can be traced back to vast and numerous studies on the subject carried out since the beginning of time. Take a look at this: if it's not true, then what is the reason why research on the subject continue to be in existence up to in the 1800s? If there's smoke and a very long-running one at that, it is a fire!

In the course of history around the world nearly every culture and civilization has been able to relate stories of its inhabitants experiencing trances and states which can be easily recognized as the state of hypnosis. China and India both of the oldest and longest long-established civilizations on Earth are home to ancient documents detailing how pains from surgery were alleviated by hypnosis when the concept of actual anesthetics was centuries away from being thought of.

As a result of this, the application of hypnosis in conjunction with surgical techniques was brought into Europe when , in 1974, Jacob Grimm (of Grimm's Fairy Tales) had a smooth recovery from a surgery to remove tumors using only the use of hypnosis (through telling stories) for anesthesia. Hypnosis was also employed to treat post-traumatic stress disorder in veterans of war.

The Placebo Reality

If there's a factor that binds both hypnosis and placebo effects in one it's the fact that both depend on the power of faith and suggestions. This means that it's virtually impossible to come up with a the illusion of control through placebo with regard to hypnotism. However that placebo effect as well as hypnotism might be the same thing.

Although the cause of the placebo effect remains to remain a mystery to scientists, research has confirmed the existence of this effect. Numerous research studies in the field of medicine were ongoing carried out where participants took medications or "medicines" which contained no active or real components (placebos) in which they were instructed on how these "medicines" could help relieve their ailments. In many instances they performed just similarly to the real medicine (placebo effects). In a few rare instances where the placebos outperformed the real drugs. Since placebos lack substance that is active they could be that the reason for the difference was what participants believed that the placebos would be able to do, which was affected by the ideas of the researchers. It is then the matter of "deceiving" our minds into believing that something is true, e.g., that placebos can be effective. What about hypnotism?

Chapter 7: History of Hypnotism

Hypnosis has been in use since antiquity and the whole concept and evolution of hypnotherapy and hypnosis could be found in old texts and documents. Hypnosis has been practiced for many centuries, but became popular only in the 18th century. According to some, the French are the very first people to discover and perfect hypnosis to turn it into an actual art form. In the 1840s, James Braid was the one who came up with the term "hypnotism. In this method, he believed that hypnosis is more focused on self-centeredness and awareness than simply captivating someone. There are numerous documents and texts that demonstrate the an importance on the hypnosis. Although many believe that the French were the founders There are a number of documents from the past, that prove otherwise.

According to historians such as Will Durant, he didn't believe that the French invented the concept of hypnotism. He believed that Indians employed hypnotism as an instrument. It was his belief that Hindus who lived throughout India had the foresight to use the art of hypnotism in a large amount. The Gurus Rishis along with other hermits engaged in meditation, concentration and concentration. This was believed to have been used to connect with Hindu Gods and Goddesses. People who were unwell in the ancient India were referred to monks who meditated in temples. The monks were able to treat the ailments and ailments of people who sought them out through the process of hypnosis. According to other sources, Avicenna from Persia identified sleep and hypnotic state. The Persian psychologist outlined the distinctions in his book , 'The Book Of Healing'. In the book, he states that hypnosis is a condition that allows a person to cause conditions and circumstances to one individual while another person accepts this as a fact.

There has also been a lot of speculation on mesmerism and magnetism in the field of hypnotism. It is believed that hypnotism originated by these two. For example, Valentine Greatrakes from Ireland was a popular figure due to his capacity to make use of magnets to heal his patients. He was known by some as "the great Irish Stroker" because of his skills. Paracelsus was a doctor from Switzerland who employed magnets to heal people that proved highly efficient. A Catholic priest named Johann Joseph Gassner healed people with hypnosis. He believed that ailments caused by evil spirits could disappear from the body by prayer and meditation. The 17th century saw the introduction of magnets father Maximilian Hell who was a Jesuit from Vienna utilized magnets by placing them on the bodies of patients to treat the ailments. One of his students were Franz Anton Mesmer, who invented modern forms of hypnosis.

Franz Anton Mesmer was an Austrian scientist who revolutionized the science of hypnosis. Mesmer studied and created something called mesmerism. It is sometimes referred to as animal magnetism. In this manner, he differentiated the traditional form of magnetism made using magnets and animal magnetism , which refers to the power that everyone possessed within the. Animals and humans could use this force to improve themselves. Influenced by the work of Richard Mead who was an English doctor, Franz Anton Mesmer discovered that when patients bled, they were able to create resistance through the use of the magnet and then passing it across the cut. The magnetic force caused that the bleeding cease. He was a huge hit in France particularly with the wealthy and powerful citizens of France due to his capacity to treat patients using magnets. It was at this time that medical professionals had to contend with him , and thus put forward an opportunity. In response to the demands from the medical community the French royals and aristocrats created the board, which included the chemist Lavoisier as well as a physician with expertise in regulating the pain of Joseph Ignace Guillotin and Benjamin Franklin. Mesmer was not willing to take part in the challenge and refused to answer any of

the questions the board posed. He instead ,
made his student the Dr. D'Eslon who
experimented on the patient. He placed the
patient in a blindfold and the results revealed
the patient's responsiveness when compared
to the tree, which has been magnetized. The
board endorsed the findings as well and
believed mesmerism can be achieved only
through imagination. Although, this type of
therapy is a different method that has gained
huge acceptance, Mesmer kept to himself and
retreated to Switzerland which is where he
later died.

Mesmer's coinage received lots of support.
There were many advocates of this type of
practice. In the French revolution mesmerism
was utilized to manage the populace. Indeed,
documents and books provide an in-depth
description of how French aristocrats
gathered people who were practicing this art.
There are theories that suggest that the social
order could be restored by mesmerism. It was
during this time that magnetism began to
fade away. People stopped using magnetism

in large quantities and moved to mesmerism. Abbe Faria, a priest from the 19th century was an Indo Portuguese priest who channeled the fascination of the public in animal magnetics. He invented what Parisians considered to be oriental hypnosis during the 18th century. He was originally from India and traveled around the globe and displayed his unique style of magnetism. He didn't utilize patients and did not confirm medical motives. He also didn't manipulate the outcomes. The primary distinction between the mesmerism method developed through Mesmer as well as Faria's Oriental hypnosis was Faria was of the opinion that powers were created by the subconscious mind of the individual. By cooperation and education individuals could project themselves more effectively and improve their abilities to think. The hypnosis techniques he used were studied, expanded and studied in detail by experts such as Hippolyte Bernheim and Ambroise-Auguste Loveault. The framework Faria created and the expansion and refinement of his theories by a variety of individuals contributed to the creation of innovative techniques such as the autogenic techniques for training that were developed in the work of Johannes Heinrich Schultz and the autosuggestion techniques that were developed in the work of Emile Coue. Marquis de Puysegur was the first to use somnambulism into the mainstream of science. It was his apprenticeship to Mesmer as well as his followers and disciples were referred to as Experimentalists. They were advocates of the Paracelsus theory. Mesmer's fluidism.

As stated earlier, the precise date of the genesis of hypnotism is not known and there are a number of documents dating back to that period in 18th century. One of them is of Recamier who practiced a particular method of hypnotism prior to its actual emergence and acclaim. He was a doctor who practiced a form of hypnotism like hypnoanesthesia, where he helped his patients heal after having them fall into a stupor. After his death, Carl Reichenbach researched extensively about the energy Recamier employed.

Although many believed that Recamier was possessed of supernatural and magical abilities, Carl Reichenbach tried to discover a scientific explanation for this energy. The energy was named after Odin, the Norse god Odin and was referred to as Odic force. The scientific community was skeptical of all Reichenbach's theories and explanations. In 1846 following the publication of the book called "The power of the Mind over the Body written of James Braid that Reichenbach's explanation was dismissed as pseudoscientific.

However, the widespread use of hypnotism was used in one form or another spread. It was a phenomenon that only occurred in the 18th century only. In actuality mesmeric sleeping was employed to treat pain in British India. India. Doctor James Esdaile operated upon about 350 patients, inducing them into a state of consciousness in a coma using mesmeric techniques. The practice was utilized prior to the introduction the chemical anesthetic. The practice was greatly decreased after the chemical anesthetic had been discovered. Hypnosis is still practiced in a few remote pockets of the globe. A surgeon named John Elliotson from England also performed this procedure. He utilized hypnosis to carry out surgeries. The procedures proved efficient and painless thanks to the use of hypnosis.

James Braid served as a surgeon, and was originally from Scotland. Braid was among the first person to create the term hypnotism. He argued for this through his work Practical Essay regarding the Curative Mechanism of Neuro-Hypnotism. It was his belief that hypnotism is something that soothed nerves and put them to sleep. His view of hypnotism was distinct from the views of mesmerists. He believed there was scientific reasons and explanations for what they believed to be an ethereal force. James Braid ridiculed mesmerists especially in their belief that their patients had powers such as telepathy and other the ability to telekinetically communicate. Braid was heavily influenced by the ideas that were a part of Scottish Common Sense Realism who believed that mesmerism was achieved through the laws of psychology and philosophy rather than religious beliefs. In the future, Braid was regarded as an hypnotist in the real sense because of his perspective of hypnotism through the psychology and physiology and not the magnetists or mesmerists.

The mesmeric trance-like condition was believed to be the physiological process that was triggered by concentration and focus on a fixed or moving object. Concentration and focus required an amount of time, put the mind of the individual to rest. The intense concentration led to fatigue of the brain, making the mind sleep and causing the state of trance.

James Braid formulated the term hypnotism derived from the Greek word meaning sleep since the hypnotist believed it originated as a result of sleep. Further research conducted by his perspective revealed the hypnotism was not an form of sleep, and Braid sought to define the phenomenon as monideism. Monoideism is the process in which one single thought or dominant thought can send the person in a state of state of trance. He believed that the trance was brought on by focus rather than sleep. The term hypnotism remained in use and was frequently employed. Neurypnology is the very first work written about the topic of hypnotism. James Braid wrote it. After his death in 1859 popular hypnotism within Britain was diminished and then it became popular in France. In France the vast research was conducted in the field of the field of hypnotism. It was during this time that the work that were written by Jean Martin Charcot and Hippolyte Bernheim gained immense acclaim.

Following the time that Braid released his book about hypnotism the author began to receive reports and letters that talked about meditation methods. Braid addressed these in a variety of articles, which he described as Magic Mesmerism, Magic, Hypnotism, etc.

The Historical Background and the Physiological Basis. There were many parallels to meditation practices used by monks and hermits as well as his opinion on the practice of hypnotism. In his articles , he shed light on the many similarities between the different spiritual practices practiced in those who practiced the Hindus in India by way of yoga, as well as other spiritual practices of India and his opinions regarding the practice of hypnotism. He was planning to incorporate meditation and broaden the scope of hypnotism. His interest increased when he was exposed to the ancient Persian documents and other texts which shed light on spiritual and religious rituals of India. One such document was the 'School Of Religions in Persia.

Within his work Braid mentions that a man from Edinburgh who lived in India wrote a letter as a response to his book. In the letter, he discusses his views and opinions regarding mesmerism, hypnotism and my personal beliefs. He further states that the person who wrote his letter described the similarities Braid's views regarding hypnotism was with traditional religious practices of the past. He suggested the Persian text , 'Dabistan', which talked about meditation and the way it aims to achieve the desired results. After reading the book, he discovered many of his beliefs and opinions that were in common with the words in the texts. The hermits and saints also used hypnosis, and performed it according to the method Braid has stated in the book. The texts also shed an understanding of the numerous advantages of self-hypnosis and meditation. But the only aspect that made the style of his writing from the techniques and writings that were outlined in the texts was that the text was of a religious in nature. A further study of the Dabistan proved that hypnosis can be performed by anyone and it did not require a third party to perform it. It can be performed on its own without the help of a professional. He drew conclusion from his book and concluded that self-hypnosis, in particular, was merely a kind of meditation and not the result of magnetism and mesmerism.

In later years, he outlined in a number of his personal stories that people who suffer from illness can enter the state of trance or even get their nerves to fall asleep, without the help of a doctor or professional hypnotist. You can achieve it by keeping an eyes and focusing on a specific area and capturing the mental energy. Spiritual and religious Persians as well as Hindus have been practicing this for centuries. There isn't any force or being external to the world to create mesmerization. Focusing on an object will improve attention and concentration specifics. The thoughts of the person performing self-hypnosis will be focused and he will have more clarity since they is unable to be distracted by any other distracting thoughts. There is no other thought that lingers or other thought will hinder them from achieving.

While there were many who were enthralled with hypnosis, and advocated for the practice of hypnosis as well as self-hypnosis, there were numerous critiques of the practice. Many religious leaders believed that hypnosis was dangerous and if it was not done correctly, it could lead to mental disorders. The person could become insane and cause people lose their sanity. But St. Thomas Aquinas did not believe in this, and said that hypnosis wasn't an act of sin. Loss of reasoning was not an act in resistance nor was it the same as a deprivation that was accompanied by a reason. In 1846, there were decrees issued by the Sacred Congregation of the Holy office and stated that it was in favor of this kind of practice when used in a legitimate way. The decree said that there are many misconceptions and myths regarding the practice of hypnotism. Once these were eliminated, it was just a method that can be beneficial, and if done correctly, it will not cause any problems.

The practice of hypnosis was used in the American Civil War. It was utilized to treat medical conditions and found to be highly efficient. It was during this time that the hypodermic needle was brought into being. It was also employed with common anesthetics such as chloroform and ether. Although hypnosis proved effective many field physicians were wary of treating patients with hypnosis. soldiers.

Jean Martin Charcot was a French neurologist who advocated for the application of hypnosis as a way to treat and prevent the condition of hysteria. He began with what became known as the 'Numerical Method', which was built on numerous experiments and tests carried out within the realm of hypnosis across various countries such as Germany, France and Switzerland. In the period of time, the light was into post-hypnosis. Numerous studies and research showed the positive relationship between hypnosis, memory enhancement and hypnosis. It is believed that hypnosis could be contributed to the improvement of the improvement of sensory ability.

It was not until the 1880s that there began to be a change in the purpose of hypnosis to being used for surgical procedures and creating uninvolved relaxation, without the use of anesthetics for surgeons to those working with mental health issues, such as psychologists or therapists. While Charcot was the person who initiated this change however, it was his student Pierre Janet who continued with this. He proposed a theory known as Dissociation theory, which dealt with separate mind and thoughts while under the influence of hypnosis. This would result in the acquisition of abilities and memories that are deep within the subconscious. Janet's research centered around the subconscious, and he discovered methods that integrate different parts that comprise the brain.

Ambroise-Auguste Loveault was the first founder of the Nancy School. The Nancy School was also his first to write about the importance of the association between a subject that wants to be hypnotized, and one who would manipulate them (hypnotizer). He proposed a suggestion for a method that relied on suggestions and demands instead of commands and orders to induce hypnosis into minds of the subject. Hippolyte Bernheim, who was regarded as an influential figure, endorsed this idea. Bernheim was also the co-founder of the Nancy school that deals with the idea of hypnosis. They both played an important contribution to the school, making it the hub for the study of hypnotherapy particularly during the late 19th century. Other reports from the 19th century were of one of the psychologists from America named William James who gave detailed descriptions of hypnosis in the book Principles of Psychology.

There were many other groups that were formed when increasing interest in hypnosis rose. The first was the first International Congress for Clinical and Experimental Hypnotism, which occurred in Paris in 1889.

Some of the most prominent figures in history in the field of hypnotism, and the people who provided the theoretical frameworks and theories of hypnotism participated as participants. The most important people were Hippolyte Bernheim, Ambroise Auguste Liebeault, Jean Martin Charcot, and Sigmund Freud. A second meeting was to be held in the year 1900, in Paris. In 1892, the Annual Conference of the BMA encouraged the use of hypnosis for an option for therapy. At this time the idea of mesmerism or animal magnetism was not given the attention it deserves and was therefore widely discredited. Although the BMA supported using hypnosis to treat medical reasons however, medical institutions, doctors and universities were not willing to admit it as a method of treatment.

The 20th century brought various hypnotists with modernistic opinions regarding the use of this practice. One of they was an French pharmacist known as Emile Coue who also served as the first founder of the New Nancy

School. He suggested a brand new form of hypnotism referred to as conscious autosuggestion, which was a type of self-help. The practice was widely recognized by the public. the practice. An additional psychiatrist in Germany Johannes Schultz merged the ideas that of Emile Coue as well as Abbe Faria. He combined meditation practices that is found in yoga with conventional hypnosis to create the concept of Autogenic training that was a variant of self-hypnosis. A American Ukraine psychologist named Boris Sidis was the apprentice of William James at the Harvard University and developed the Law of Suggestion. In his law, he proposed that our conscious is split and becomes unification. The conscious and the subconscious are separated and the degree of this is dependent on the degree of the degree of suggestibility. Gustave Le Bon founded crowd psychology in the 20th century. In his work, he developed the concept of a parallel between the leader and the crowd. The leader is an hypnotist and his ideas influence the followers. This concept was derived from the concept of suggestibility developed by Boris Sidis.

Another major contributor to the study of the field of hypnotism is Sigmund Freud. By the end of nineteenth century, the practice of hypnotism was popular. Charcot made it a popular practice and people became aware of the practice. It was the basis for the psychoanalysis of Sigmund Freud who was the pupil of Charcot. He was also influenced by the numerous experiments carried out by Hippolyte Berheim and Liebeault at the Nancy School. In this way, he worked together with Josef Breuer and formulated the abreaction treatment using the hypnosis method. He utilized this technique as part of his experiments, and further developed the use of hypnosis in the field of psychiatry. It was a way for many psychiatrists used hypnotism.

Obstetric hypnosis, which is a type of hypnosis that was extensively utilized throughout Russian healthcare practices. Platanov was one of the most famous Russian medical doctor, became famous because of his frequent use of hypnoobstetric as a method of curing. The result was a number of instances of success that caught the interest of Stalin. Stalin created a national program based on this. The program was headed by Velvoski and brought together the methods used by Pavlov in hypnosis and the hypno-obstetrical principles of Platanov. Others like Fernand Lamaze developed the application of the hypnosis method. He travelled to Russia during the 19th century after the use of hypnosis was gaining popularity due to an uproar in Russia. He brought the idea of unhurried childbirth to France and the reflexology process was with hypnotic ideas and utilized psychological techniques.

In the 20th century, we also witnessed the rise of hypnosis and hypnotherapy throughout wartime. For World War I, Korean Wars, World War II and other wars it was utilized as a basis to treat neuroses. It was incorporated with the theories of psychiatry and was widely used for treating Post

Traumatic Stress Disorder. It achieved a wide range of successful rates. William McDougall was psychologist from England who treated soldiers as well as the military from the hypnosis. He dealt with issues such as acute trauma and shocks. He also was not a proponent of Freudian theories, particularly aspects such as abreaction, which was a commonly utilized concept in Freudian theory.

The British developed an Act known as"the Hypnotism Act in 1952. The act protected against illegal conduct of those who hypnotize. The act was aimed at regulating the activities of hypnotizers to serve entertainment for entertainment purposes. In 1955, the British Medical Association advocated hypnosis. They endorsed the use of hypnotic techniques in areas like hypnoanesthesia as well as psychoneuroses. It was employed to manage of pain, particularly in situations such as childbirth or surgery. It was during this time that all doctors and medical doctors were required to undergo a basic course in the art of hypnosis.

Study of the hypnotist phenomenon was first conducted in the 1920s. One of the pioneers in this field is Clark Leonard Hull who was psychologist at Yale University. Hull employed statistics and then paired it with analysis to investigate the hypnotic phenomena that were a result of numerous experiments. He documented this in his paper called 'Hypnosis & Suggestibility'. The results of his research and experiments showed that sleep and hypnosis are two distinct aspects. Actually, hypnosis has no link to sleep and there were many myths surrounding sleep and the hypnosis. Clark Hull aimed at busting myths and debunking the myths surrounding the hypnosis process. He concentrated on the advantages of the practice of hypnosis. His research showed that people who were hypnotized experienced an increase in their performance as they could concentrate more effectively and clearly. They also showed an increase in their cognitive performance. The entire research conducted by Hull shed light on the substantial reduction in pain experienced by patients who were hypnotized and the way they experienced improvements of their memories. Hull took an approach that was based on behavior to hypnosis. His work proved that these things can occur without the aid of hypnosis. If you combine the power of suggestion, motivation and encouragement the hypnosis process works better. Physical limitations and any shifts in sensations can be translated into a psychological.

Andrew Salter who introduced it to the American people. The masses embraced the Pavalovian method of the hypnosis. This technique was designed to combat the opposition, contradiction and challenge of traditional beliefs and values. He combined the principles of hypnosis using a technique known as classical conditioning. The idea was influenced by Ivan Pavlov who also experimented with hypnotism , and changed the mental state of pigeons to "Cortical inhibition".

Up until the 20th century, until the 20th century, Roman Catholic Church banned hypnotism. It was only in late 20th century that the pope Pius XII gave the green signal to the practice of hypnotism. However, he also said that hypnosis was only permissible for legal purposes, such as diagnosis and medical facilities. It is used in medical procedures by medical professionals. It may also be utilized for childbirth however it is important to exercise caution. It was the Pope considered that the practice of hypnotism is something that shouldn't be used unless understood correctly. Only ethically-sound practices are permitted, and only those who have a strong moral values can engage in it. If it is utilized as an anesthetic , the rules for different forms of anesthetics will apply to the practice of hypnotism. Similar to that it is the case that American Medical Association also approved the use of hypnosis for medical reasons. The organization promoted research and study into the use of hypnosis, but discouraged some aspects of hypnosis which they felt were not adequately studied and thus could lead to issues. In the early days, even the American Psychological Association approved hypnosis and recognized it as an area of psychology. Following it was the Second World War, there were more studies conducted. Sarbin, Hilgard, Barber and Orne made contributions to the study of hypnotism. Stanford Scales were widely used in the year 1961. Andre Muller Weitzenhoffer and Ernest Hilgard developed the scale that measures the level of vulnerability people are to hypotheses. This scale was employed to draw conclusions from different genders and age groups. Of them, Hilgard pursued his studies and research into the induced anesthesia sensory deception, analgesia and sensory deception.

Harry Arons was a person who contributed to the spread of the practice of the hypnotism technique. He was able to do this by initiating professional classes and training in various cities across the US. A large number of psychiatrists, doctors and physiologists were educated by his teachings. Training sessions that ran over forty years in which people were taught the many applications of the hypnosis. He was also one of the most influential individuals who could convince medical professionals to utilize the hypnosis method. His fifty years of expertise in the field helped him become a household name. This is the reason that doctors often attended his conferences and lectures. He joined the faculty of the National Academy of Medicine Hypnosis and also served as editor, writer, and editor. He also served as a consultant and permitted psychotherapists, psychologists, psychiatrists and dentists to speak with him and offer them medical advice on the practice of hypnosis. He also worked with individuals like Ki Ho Kim, Harold Hansen and Samuel Martin to name a few. He was editor of Hypnosis Quarterly and published a number of books on hypnosis. Some of his most renowned books were 'Handbook for Professional Hypnosis as well as "New Master Course in Hypnotism'. He also advocated the use of hypnotism to treat criminals and wrote "Hypnosis for Criminal Investigation". Arons, who travelled extensively to promote this method instructed law police agencies. Famous attorneys and lawyers were also taught by him. He was a mentor, teacher and guide , who helped the community to accept his work and recognize the practice of hypnosis. He tried to extend the field of hypnosis and expand its use in courts and trails. In his time, he established the Association to Advance Ethics in Hypnosis following his stint as the director of the International Society for Professional Hypnosis.

Most often, it was the spreading of hypnosis in the medical field. Dave Elman was another person who promoted hypnosis to promote this purpose. He taught dentists and doctors on the practice of hypnotism even though the fact that he was not medical professional. He was the first to define hypnotism. It is the definition he gave that is extensively employed. He pioneered rapid inductions and it is now the most commonly used type of Hypnotism. He also shed the light on the hypnotic coma. This time period also saw the rise of stage hypnotists as well as the creation of the profession of hypnotherapist. One of them was Ormond McGill, who was also serving as dean of the American Hypnotists, and also published numerous studies.

Skills for Health, the government's Sector Skills Council for the UK health sector, published an hypnotherapy-specific book known as National Hypnotherapy Standards for Occupational Practices in 2002. Courses and training were offered and even certificates courses and diplomas awarded through the Qualifications and Curriculum Authority. There were international conferences organized and tests were conducted, and those who performed very well were awarded medals. In India the practice of hypnotism is employed for a number of years. Since 2003, the Ministry of Health & Family Welfare, Government of India declared in one of the letters it released that hypnotherapy was a viable option. It is a method to treat patients, but only for ethical reasons with a certified hypnotist. Nowadays, it is utilized to alleviate pain after birth, surgeries as well as mental health and other issues.

Chapter 8: Types of Hypnotism

The next step is to continue to process, as we've learned the fundamentals of putting the subject in the state of hypnotic trance and learning new methods.

James Braid's Eye Fixation Method:

The method, which is one of the most widely-used is also known as Braidism. There have been quite variety of modifications that have been made to this method in order to arrive at the present eye-fixation methods, such as the method of induction employed in the Stanford Hypnotic Susceptible Scale or SHSS which is the most commonly utilized research tool in hypnotic field.

If you stare up at the sky without any head movement, and you concentrate on any aspect of what you see You may be experiencing hypnosis, which can be sleep-inducing.

Upward looking is stressful and can increase the strain on the eyes. Don't move your head forward to this point as this assists the eyes and relieves strain on the eyes. Only turn your eyes, but not your head. Keep it in the same way as your neck.

In the event that your eyes stay stable in this place, you will not feel any strain on your eyes. You will more likely feel like you are sleeping. While you're in the process of hypnosis, you'll experience an intense state of mind as you focus your eyes on one spot.

To get the subject to follow James Braid's method select a brightly lit object, which is ideally using a lancet case or something similar, that is placed on the thumb of your left middle finger and fore. Holding the object that is illuminated around 8 to 10 inches away from the eyes in a location in which the subject is likely to put in the most effort to keep his eyes at the object. The hypnotist should ensure that the subject's attention is focused only the object that is in his hands in order to make the technique work efficiently.

It is essential to ensure that the patient comprehends the fact that co-operation is crucial to the success of the procedure that is why he needs to maintain his focus upon the object in the hypnotist's hands. If the object is carefully engulfs the subject then it is observed that the following things happen. The first noticeable change could be the shrinking of the pupil in the subject due to the acclimatization process that is consensual to the eye . This constriction gradually turns into dilation. The hypnotist has now decided to disengage the object from the subject's gaze, and replace the object with their own. The subject is to shut his eyes, but involuntarily this signals that the subject is entering the hypnotic trance.

There is a chance that your subject will not allow you to induce a stupor, and blames it on the lack of concentration. In these instances it is our obligation to make him realize the significance of his immersion in the object and ensure that he keeps his attention on the object, and not elsewhere. In general the subject will go through the trance without obstruction.

Arm Drop Method:

The name says its own, the arm drop technique of induction is a technique in which the relationship between the hypnotist's subject and the subject, and the efficacy is determined through the control of the subject on his arms.

At first the subject is instructed to raise his arm over his head. Be sure that the arm is not resting on anything and is able to be lowered with a touch. The hypnotist could then start talking to the subject, permitting him to enter a semi-conscious state of trance.

What a hypnotist should perform during the course of their work is a throbbing question. After ensuring that the arm is properly positioned before hypnotizing, the hypnotist will begin to formulate his suggestions. We request the person to for him to concentrate his gaze on one finger on the arm that is elevated. Then we speak to him, insisting that he focus completely upon the fingers. We could also offer suggestions to him on psychological aspects that are meant to make him feel comfortable and light. When he is focused on a particular finger on his arm, the person could feel other fingers become black. While he's completely immersed in his gaze, fixed on his finger as the arm begins to lower it self. We should note that the more the arm falls the close the subject is being attracted to the experience.

From the perspective of the subject the experience is interesting. It is a unique experience. the one of a kind. When the subject is focused and more focused on their finger, the hand elevated is a feeling of being more and more heavy.

However, it's considered that the hypnotist is merely expressing what he perceives, rather than what he expects or anticipates to occur. For example, the person who hypnotizes might say to the person "Now you can feel your arm dropping" as the subject actually feels the arm dropping , not because he anticipates the arm to fall.

Arm Levitation method:

This method of induction demands not just the focused determination of the individual but also the meticulously monitored speed with which he makes suggestions to the subject.

The perfect conversation or ideas to discuss the subject, are similar to these. They begin "As I count from one to twenty-five A mild tickle sensation will begin to creep through your left arm, and then continue to move through it. The fingers will move around, without notice, and without conscious effort. When you finally let go of the feeling, instead of trying to control your feelings and feel completely liberated, you'll see your arm rise over your body. It will rise, over the level of your body but not when you attempt to feel self-conscious, and not in the event that you control your thoughts and control, but only when you release the deepest feelings that are in you!"

The most important thing to keep with you is the fact that the hypnotist is always able to insist, but not oblige the subject. It is crucial that in this manner, the level of authority at which the hypnotist gives instructions on the person being instructed. The hypnotist should continue to suggest an idea only after ensuring that the subject is aware of the previously mentioned points.

Relaxation technique:

It is among the most commonly employed techniques. The fundamentals of this technique are practically nonexistent apart from the confidence you create in the subject's mind. The method is based on the voice tone and the words spoken by the hypnotist in order for the subject to go in a state of induced hypnosis. Therefore, the hypnotist has to be calm and soothing, instead of domineering and in control. As hypnotists, we try to make the puddle of emotions and focus on the ones that need to be taken care of and to do this the person being hypnotized must be persuaded to let his guard down. You won't be able to let your guard down unless you can trust him. This, in turn is the most important aspect to accomplish when using this method of introduction.

As hypnotists, we may employ a polite yet confident tone to help the person trust us, not only in a conscious way but as well subconsciously. Instruct him to recall all the fun and jolly memories and then that he is gradually surrendering to the sub-conscious. If he's completely relaxed, we will tell him to be aware of your breath, and feel the blood flow through his body.

The method is to treat the subject as an active participant in the process. That is it allows the hypnotist to perform all the work, and the subject simply listens and is obligated to him in full. The technique employs relaxation as a technique to induce hypnosis, however it is slightly different from the earlier one.

Instead of being acting as a passive observer instead, he becomes actively participating in this method. In this case, the hypnotist suggests that that is relaxed the extremities of his body are loose and soft as well as sloppy and limp as if the stuffed doll made of cloth. Then, raise their hand and suggest that they allow the entire adiposity of your arm hang from your fingers. After a while , drop it, letting your subject feel a calming sensation across his entire arm. Encourage him to spread the waves throughout your body, rubbing his body from head to the toe.

Repeat the process by the opposite hand and with the same hand for a long time until the user is in a Trance. While he's already in a state of calm however, he may feel the intensity of relaxation increasing dramatically through this method. These two strategies could be utilized in conjunction, as in employing the first method to relax him and the other to get him into the state of semi-consciousness.

Staircase method:

Hypnotismat its essence, is a journey by the thin line that separates the physical photoreceptors as well as the imagined photoreceptors. The imaginary or, in other words the eyes of the mind can be described as the eyes that give form to our thoughts and our imaginations. Hypnosis being one of the psychological sciences is more appealing to the imaginative view than to the physical eyes. This is one method of appeal.

The staircase method is like in all methods that is unflappable and calm concentration is maintained, uninfluenced from the surrounding environment. The hypnotist is able to calm down the subject and lets the subject relax with eyes shut. The hypnotist then informs to the subject that he's going to count numbers. He should also explain to the person to keep in mind that while counting the numbers from lower to higher it is necessary to imagine him going down the stairs. When the hypnotist has completed all of his count the subject is urged to imagine falling onto a bed or into a pool, and then sink further and farther into bed, or pool.

It symbolically represents the state of mind for the individual. When he is at peace The descending of the stairs is in sync with the process of getting deeper into the thoughts of the subject. In this, the initial few steps of the staircase represent the most superficial, topmost thinking of the individual and the last few steps represent the most profound insidemost, hidden thoughts that have been forgotten by the subject.

The subject is thought to be completely the trance, and only when they have reached the end of the pool that he's thrown himself in.

Association Method:

This is of the methods that are widely utilized. This is one of the techniques that are based on the trustworthiness that the subject has on the hypnotist as well as the trust that the hypnotist established in the subconscious of the individual. The essence of this technique is the hypnotist's diligent and arduous efforts by the subject to comply with the suggestions of the hypnotist. If at any time during or prior to the procedure does the subject not follow the directions of the hypnotist outcomes are not likely to be successful. Therefore, it is essential that the hypnotist can exert a powerful but subtle influence over the subject's unconscious. Be sure to ensure that the hypnotist is only in possession of the physical presence, not the authority. This means that the hypnotist has the power to guide or suggest the actions the subject may take and possibly feel, and not force, coerce or force him to feel or do this way, and not for any reason other than simply because "It does not work this way". The following paragraph could provide insight into the hypnotist's perspective on using the method of association.

In this case, as a hypnotist we nudge the subject out of their minds, but not at their wishes. We make them to enter a hypnotic trance in order we can trigger the long-held feelings the person is seeking assistance in unraveling. We dig up the memories, remove them from the dust and determine what the subject wants to do with these memories. If he wishes to improve the memories, or is hoping to prevent them from surfacing and again, or if he's completely unaware of them; we uncover the entire thing. For that reason it's of no benefit to communicate with the conscious mind of the subject because it is the person who is seeking help initially. Therefore we try to calm them down, and then lure them into calm and seek out the answers inside the person. The following are the most important conversations the hypnotist should engage in with the person in question.

"Please sit comfortably." Instruct them to lie down, or sit, or be flattened however it suits them. "Now as you slide into a state of unconsciousness Please pay attention to what I say" Start to explain to themon what to not do instead of the things to be done in order to ensure that they follow your ideas and words. "Please be aware that you're in this place to relax and not be stifled in letting go. Therefore, consider sleeping and don't limit your desires. Accept them as they are to see what can help you. Do not retaliate when you feel the urge that you're letting it go. Take off the weights and focus on what is bothering you." When you speak you could also observe the breathing patterns of the subject shift to a more relaxed style and this is when they are entering an euphoric state. induced and this is when we as hypnotists can unravel the memory and assist the subject to get the information they require.

Method for misdirection:

What can you do with kids who don't want to hear you? What if they don't want to pay to eat chocolate? What happens if they're sufficiently mature to read however they are not too childish to play with toys? This is a level that a subject's subconscious could reach. They do not think about it however, subconsciously try to avoid or avoid being in a state of hypnosis. What can we do?

Reverse psychology may be a colloquial term used to describe it. The technical term is misdirection. It is when we take people completely off the notion of hypnotism and take the audience off guard. That's right. As the guard is lower, it gets complicated, it makes people not think about it in all.

To achieve this it is necessary to keep them interested and engaged. Let them be able to answer every questions and keep their minds busy. Ask them what they can picture as an image in their minds. For instance, imagine yourself driving, swimming or sitting in the front porch sipping tea. Ask them to write down the imagined scenarios, for example the event that they imagined themselves driving, ask whether they can actually describe the route they were driving on, and ask them if they could see any trees on the sides or if they were by themselves or had anyone else present when they drove. Also , ask them if were the only driver on the road. If they weren't, ask them to describe the cars travelling along. Ask whether they can identify the inside of the vehicle that they were driving. This includes the color of the interiors as well as the side on which the steering wheel was. We're more concerned with distracting them from the notion of being hypnotized. But we should inquire as many times as we can.

If they had imagined themselves in their front porch, it would be simple for them to answer the question about the hue of the house, as it is a normal thing for them to be aware of the hue of the paint. It is more beneficial to question them about the smallest specifics, to remain as active as it is possible. For example, ask whether the neighbor's house has mailboxes, and in the absence of neighbors, ask them about the location. In the end, ensure that they are engaged to a certain extent.

If you're confident that they're not worried about getting hypnotized then it's time to ramp it up. Encourage them to rolling their eyes to focus and gaze into the dark and then focus in your middle eyebrows and in their foreheads. in some cases it's even fine to give a gentle pressure or rub their foreheads to aid them in concentrating better. Tell them to lifting their eyes, without turning their eyes away from the darkness. They will feel their lids locking tighter. The more they attempt to open their eyes and close them, the more tightly they seal. This is why you instruct them to ease off and let their body feel stiff and to let them feel their breathing and the flow of blood. It is apparent that they fall into a state of trance.

The use of hypnosis in children

Do you wonder what the reason is that children require hypnotization? The following paragraphs can aid you in understanding. In essence, it's more comfortable to sit on a mat than standing on the needle. So, the more expansive the field of view the less awkward and cluttered the mind is. Also, since children are they are so isolated from their world their minds are extremely tightly woven and are much more effort-intensive than adult minds. Children aren't able to comprehend changes as easily as adults do and , therefore, you must make them believe that there has taken place no changes. There are many problemsin this adorable world they live in. From mental traumas to bedwetting there are plenty of problems that children experience for which there aren't medications for physical use. That's why they'll require therapy with hypnosis. The methods and techniques used are quite liberal. We gently, gently transport them into a state of trance and then let them experience a relaxed and comfortable. The method we employ to induce children into hypnosis is called known as the "Bionic Arm Method".

The bionic arm is the most commonly used method used by children. Guess what children love? Stories! Yay! That's what we're planning to do! Let them know about the man who had an arm that was stiff! It's difficult to tell the children since they are not keen on what is known as the Bionic Arm Method of Induction which helps the person be in a hypnotic state. They are attracted by stories. Therefore, we inform them about the Bionic method that we are interested in, by telling a story that they are keen on.

In the first place, ask whether they know the tale! They don't, but offer the boy a few minutes. When they're ready, begin talking to them about the man with that right arm. Inform them that their right arm looks exactly as the man's! Tell them that the man was lying on a mattress, comfy and relaxed, exactly as they are today. Also, consider them in comparison to the fictional character and are in the place as the right-handed man.

Tell them that one day his arm stiffened! It was as stiff as an old baseball bat! Try it out for the dramatics They might enjoy it! Inform them that the more they attempted to loosen the arm, the more stiff it got. It is possible that kids are trying to loosen their arms as well, but they're too stiff to allow them to move. Keep telling them that the arm is getting stiffer and more, until eventually the arm is completely lump and relax , and a feeling of relaxation flows across the arm. Let their arms relax. Then tell them to spread the waves across their body, and make their body extremely at ease. Then, tell them to imagine the things that bother them. Ask them to describe the issue, and there we begin! We've successfully hypnotized our big guy!

The next major question:

The next major issue is: Do my child really require to be controlled by a hypnotist?

There are a variety of reasons why children may experience traumas for example,

Unsafe or unstable atmosphere

Separation from an adult

A serious illness

Medical procedures that are not intrusive

Physical, sexual or verbal abuse

Domestic violence

Neglect

Bullying

Children are fragile, light and immeasurablely pure and sturdy. It is very easy for them to break by the fragility of them, however it's hard for us to understand what caused them to break because it is protected within their more robust skin. The child is not the type to tell you that he's being harassed or struggling with his sleeping habits. It's almost impossible to understand this for ourselves until we get into them, and for that using hypnosis is the most effective and sole method.

Hypnosis is a highly effective method to treat a range of problems that children face. As opposed to adults, children are typically more open to hypnosis due to the fact that they have a higher level of suggestibility. Children have vivid imaginations which allow them to reach the unconscious and create the desired changes. Therefore the use of hypnosis in children can yield rapid results. Hypnotists can employ various techniques for children such as visualization, stories as well as puppets, role-playing and other games.

Children are excellent subjects for hypnosis as they aren't subject to the same years of resistance and conditioning that adults do. Since they have a background of learning, they are usually more willing to try something new, for example, the use of hypnosis. Children aren't as likely to be skeptical about the process. These factors make it easy for a hypnotist deal with children. Adults however tend to be cautious or even hesitant and could be conscious and subconscious resistance to being attracted to hypnosis. It doesn't mean they won't be hypnotized; it's possible that it won't happen with the same ease.

Hypnosis can be a successful treatment for a variety of issues, concerns and disorders among children. The most common ones are learning issues such as anxiety, academic performance and self-esteem issues, bedwetting and homework battles as well as thumb sucking and fear of dark. Additionally, dealing with traumatizing events such as the loss of a parent or having parents divorced are issues that can be solved by the use of hypnosis. Children who experience frequent nightmares might benefit from hypnosis as well. Hypnosis may also make children less nervous in the event of a surgical procedure, such as surgery.

School is a huge area of struggle for many youngsters. Everything from learning to homework problems to conflicts with other children can be resolved by the help of hypnotherapy. Most often, just two or three sessions are required to get efficient outcomes. Children can experience significant improvement in confidence and the capability to achieve success by using the power of hypnosis. Hypnosis is a great way to help them develop healthy and effective coping strategies. It helps to enhance and unleash their creative potential. With the assistance from a good hypnotist children can truly grow and become more productive and happy.

Hypnosis to stop bedwetting has been proven to be successful with a lot of children. Children who have a problem with bedwetting frequently struggle with shame and embarrassment. They also suffer from a insecurity. They are often vulnerable and their self-esteem could be severely damaged if the issue isn't addressed and solved promptly. One of the reasons why Hypnosis could be a beneficial solution to this particular problem in childhood is the fact that the subconscious mind is responsible for controlling most of the bodily activities. Hypnosis taps into the unconscious mind and uses a combination of visualization and suggestion to stop the process of bedwetting.

Your child can listen to a CD of hypnosis designed to treat bedwetting. You can also use techniques of hypnosis to help your child. It is usually best to seek out the hypnotist prior to consulting. Any method can be effective in basically reprogramming your child's mind to respond to the necessity of going to the bathroom even when he's asleep, just like he does while awake.

It is possible to help your child to relax by sitting comfortably in a chair , where there is peace and quiet, and where there aren't any distractions. A low-lighting environment is advantageous. It can help your child to relax by having him shut your eyes while taking deep, slow breaths. Encourage him to consider the object of his choice or ask him to imagine the place where he is at ease and secure. If your child is agitated, you must keep your cool so that he can calm down.

If your child seems comfortable, you can make affirmative, encouraging statements about the issue of bedwetting. Some suggestions for statements that could be used to assist with bedwetting might include "You can keep your bladder in check throughout your entire evening" as well as "You always get up whenever you feel that you need to use toilet". After saying these words several times, you will be able to get your child back into an alert and fully aware state. The practice of having him count to ten is a good way to accomplish this. Discuss the exercise and allow him to talk about his thoughts and thoughts.

Children are extremely receptive to the hypnosis. It can be an extremely enjoyable and positive experience for children. Be sure to select the hypnotist that is competent and confident in working with children.

The taboo is that child can be hypnotized, could be as dangerous like black magic. We aren't the pips of Hamlin! We are professional psychologists. It is completely and safe for your child to be controlled. The best method to tackle the issue is to investigate the issue immediately, rather than letting it grow. A stitch can make nine! Also, you'll be required to address your child's issues when he is a kid instead of attending it once it has become unmanageable in the adult or found adult level. The issue that is bothering the child may cause permanent issues like a lower self-esteem, stammering and so on. Therefore, it's important to address the issue earlier!

Chapter 9: How to Hypnotize Someone

In this chapter , we will explore the technical aspects of how to make someone hypnotize. The act of hypnotizing someone is typically element of magic shows and frequently, we are captivated by it. In this article we will look at how you can induce hypnosis on people. Hypnotism is often conflated with spiritualism or considered as a part or a part of the spiritual. It isn't the case. Hypnotism is a method of building mental power and focusing on achieving results.

1. Choosing the Subject

The first step to hypnotize anyone is to locate an individual who would like to be attracted to you. If you're just beginning your journey it is essential to locate someone who is willing to be attracted. Be sure to inform whomever you choose to tell them what you intend to do in complete detail. Build confidence in the person by interacting with the person and making them feel feel comfortable. At the end you should feel confident of your capabilities and feel comfortable enough. They should also feel like they're in good in their hands, which can lead to greater outcomes. When choosing a person to work with, pick one who is calm and calm about the whole process. Avoid attempting to hypnotize anyone without their permission. Don't practice your skills on those suffering from issues, especially mental disorders. Hypnotism is focused on the mind, and those suffering from mental illnesses can become afflicted and cause difficult and complicated issues.

The majority of people have extremely skewed opinions about the practice of hypnotism. This is because there isn't enough information that is given to this art form via mediums like novels, movies and television shows. Hypnosis is a method which is used to relax the minds of individuals. It brings clarity and insight to the individual. It also eases the mind and eases the stress associated when you are pondering issues within the subconscious. Hypnotism is something that is a part of our lives. Actually "spacing out" is very the entirety of what hypnotism's about. And we can experience these through dreams too. It is essential to inform those you plan to hypnotize that they're not going into an unconscious state or go into a state of unconsciousness. Individuals who are hypnotized retain control over their lives and aren't under anyone other's hands. Hypnosis can have many benefits, including decreasing anxiety and increasing metabolism. It can make your mind more efficient by increasing its focus and sharp. It also boosts concentration, and acts as a method of relaxation. It is important to figure out the reason your partner would like to be attracted to you. This will help to reduce confusion, and allow you to follow through with the demand. This also gives you a opportunity to meet them and gain an understanding of their thoughts. This will make it easier to put them in a stupor like state.

Make it a priority to inquire about any experience they've had in relation to the practice of hypnotism. Learn about their thoughts about this practice and more. If they've been hypnotized , you can learn about the degree of responsiveness they showed and what made them feel uncomfortable. You can stay clear of the activities they do not want to do and choose alternative methods. You can also assess the person and partner that you're working with. It is also much easier to manipulate people who have experienced hypnotization previously. Make sure you reassure your target. They must trust your abilities and trust in the work you do. Let them be guided gently and be ready to answer every question they have.

Alongside selecting a subject to hypnotize, make sure you choose the right place. The space you choose should be free of distractions. It should be quiet and clean. It should also be relaxing. Get rid of any distracting items such as TVs, music systems , and close all windows when there's a lot of background noise. Turn off all mobiles and alarms. Lock the room and make sure that the lights are not on. It is crucial to remember that the room shouldn't be dim and dark. Be sure that it's only the two of you. Sit them comfortably in chairs.

2. Make them fall into Trance Like state

Relax them and when they have found a relaxed position and relaxed, ask them to close their eyes. Use a slow and quiet voice. Keep your voice steady and calm. Make your sentences as if you are drawing them so that they sound natural and sound like you're trying to soothe people. Make sure you speak in a soft and clear manner. It is crucial to maintain the soft, mellow tone throughout the entire hypnosis process. Instruct them to enter the zone by imagining positive moments. Alternately , you could start the process by having them picture yourself in a serene location. A lush garden , a serene meadow or something that feels calm and peaceful. Think like you would speak to your child. Make it a goal to frequently assure them. Ask them to do something rather than telling them. Inform them that they have control and that they are secure. Also , give them the time and space to follow through to your demands and suggestions. Request them to take a break as they breathe in deeply. Encourage them to focus and concentrate on a particular aspect and breathe slowly and deeply. They should be in charge for their breath. It's good to assist them in this process by matching your breathing with theirs. Make clear and concise instructions like "Take your breath in deeply and keep it in for a couple of seconds, then slowly release it". Spend a minute or two on arranging their breathing. This will improve focus and clarity due to the high levels of oxygen which will be delivered to the brain of the subject.

If you would prefer to work in a room with your subjects eyes wide, simply ensure they focus or pay attention to a particular area. Allow them to look and focus their attention on you or another object around them. It will take a while until they're focusing completely upon the thing. Be sure to keep your eye on them too. This will tell you the moment their focus is slipping. It is also possible to offer advice whenever they are distracted and gently return them to the point of concentration. Instruct them to concentrate and be attentive. Also, tell them to ease their eyelids.

When it comes to relaxation, it is crucial to let their body relax gradually. You must ensure that they are in a calm state and breathing correctly. Begin by gently instructing them to ease their feet. Request them to let their muscles and let them ease them. Continue to move towards the ceiling, like their calves their legs, their torsos shoulders, back, arms, neck and then the face. As you do this, make sure your voice remains cool and soft. Don't rush them , and allow them plenty of time to rest. Offer encouraging words and encouragement when they need it. It is essential to ensure that they're relaxed and that they feel comfortable.

Pay attention to the body language of the person and their breathing. This can give you an understanding of their state of mind. The objective at this point is to make sure your subject is relaxed and calm. If they seem rigid and uneasy, try using gentle words, soothing images, and even music that soothes them. Check for signs of the twitching and fidgeting of the eyes, such as a dar in the direction of eyes, wiggling of the toes or tapping of fingers, and other such things. If they exhibit any of these, you can help them to relaxed. You can also offer appealing scents such as incense sticks which will aid to get them into a state of relaxation more quickly.

When they're completely at ease and are been relaxed, you can begin with inducing thoughts. You could use the technique of hypnotic staircase. This is a frequent technique employed by hypnotists and hypnotherapies. It allows one to go into a trance-like state. Then ask them to imagine sitting on the top of a stairwell. Then ask them to imagine themselves walking one step at a time. Each step will cause them to relax and sink into a state of trance. The subject will become more immersed in him or her. Make use of a calm tone of voice that is controlled to achieve this. Encourage them to relax at the end of each step, providing specific instructions, such as "You are standing on top of a long staircase. you're about to begin going down this stairs, and with each step , you will be able to relax. Begin with the first step and you'll be able to feel your body relax after which, slowly step down the next step and you'll notice your mind getting relaxed." Make sure they are completely at ease and are in a trance state at the end of the exercise. It is also possible to trigger thoughts by having them move into a pleasant environment and in a peaceful location. Provide them with more information and explain the scenario clearly to allow them to visualize the scenarios in their mind's eye. Additionally, let them imagine. When they are in the state of tracing Ask them questions that describe the natural world. Ask their opinion on what color the flowers in their garden look like, which color clothing they wear and the list goes on. It will be possible to visualize what is happening in their minds by doing this exercise. After an hour or so, you'll no longer be asking them questions, but instead helping them focus their minds and make vibrant colors and shapes. Ask them to describe what they're seeing around them . When you receive clear and descriptive answers, you will know they are in a state of trance.

From this point, you can choose a more authoritative tone. Make sure your voice is soft and gentle, however, once they've entered a state of trance, you should make your voice more assertive and instructive. Instead of asking them to start the ask, try using phrases like "Do This" rather than "Could you do this". Then they'll begin to respond to you and following your instructions. They must be able to respond to your questions and completing tasks you give them instructions on. It is crucial not to ask them questions about personal issues or topics they aren't at ease discussing.

Additionally, when they are in a Trance state, utilize the positive language to stay in the state. Set a goal and stick to it. Make sure you are positive.

3. Have a Goal in Mind

You can hypnotize someone with good intent. Be sure to have a goal to achieve. It is likely that the person you're hypnotizing won't recall the things they were told to say or do. That's why it is not a good idea to break the ethical codes. You can ask them to perform easy tasks and to answer questions they'd be content to answer in the absence of hypnosis. Don't use hypnosis in order to trick or prank someone. Hypnosis is a form of art which is employed for positive reasons. As an example, for instance, you could make use of hypnosis to lower the level of anxiety in your subjects. It isn't necessary to give instructions to your students or force them to complete any job. The process of bringing them into the trance-like state has been known to lower stress levels and increase clarity. This is due to the profound relaxation they experience during the trance state. Be aware that you cannot solve any issue or any issue, however you can relax their tensions. If the person you are talking to has a specific problem, then encourage them to think of solutions. They can be encouraged to resolve their own issues instead of feeding them spoon-feeding. If, for instance, they're worried over their prospects, encourage them to imagine an improved future. You can ask them a few questions that will lead to solutions.

If they have more serious problems that you as a novice, are unable to solve then it is best to take them to an expert or an psychotherapist. If they're suffering from emotional trauma, self-esteem issues or other issues it is best to refer them to a medical specialist. If it's moderate and you're trying to convince them to stop doing something, like smoking, for instance, you're trying to convince them to stop smoking. You can then use positive words while in a trance state to help them quit smoking. Let them envision a world free of addiction by using positive words, positive imagery and soothing sounds. It's an excellent idea to understand the purpose of the person being hypnotized and why the person wants to be attracted. You can modify your technique appropriately.

Hypnotherapy is a method of relaxation. It is a method that combines relaxation and focus to achieve the best results. It is important to remember that hypnosis isn't something which is used to fix issues. It allows the person to contemplate their problems and then fix it of their own way. As a hypnotist, you can only act as a facilitator to facilitate this. Don't expect instant results. It's a slow but constant process and must be accomplished with the consent of the subject. Because it requires an enormous amount of mental power, self-reflection and reflection It is recommended to use hypnosis on someone who has an unbalanced mind. If they need help, it is recommended to refer them to an expert.

4. Completing the Hypnosis

It is essential to gradually get them out of the trance state. Avoid uttering abrupt movements or instructions. Slowly let them come from the trance and be aware of their surroundings. The most effective way to do this is to explain slowly that you'll count until a certain number , after which they will have escaped the trance-like state. While doing this, make sure to give enough pauses, at least one minute between every count. This will increase awareness. Alternately , you can lead them back to the upstairs room every step they make increasing their awareness. In this way, you can inform them that they will become more conscious and alert with a calm way. Allow them to rest and concentrate their minds once they've got up. Avoid engaging them in a lengthy conversation or ask them to complete anything demanding or tiring as this can cause confusion as well as brain fog.

If they appear to be more relaxed and stable, you can go to have a conversation with them.

Reward them and say that they performed well. Discuss the hypnosis experience with them. Have them share their thoughts and opinionsabout the way they felt, what they felt, and the list goes on. This will help you comprehend the technique more effectively and you'll be able to assess the impact of your hypnosis on someone. This will give you an understanding of the experiences of the individual and offer suggestions for corrective actions and ways to improve your skills in the art of hypnosis. Do not over-pressurize anyone, and give the person enough time to gather their thoughts. If they prefer to be left to themselves follow their request. Prepare to answer all your questions with a clear mind.

5. Answer all Queries

There is a chance that you will be confronted with an abundance of questions following your time completed using illusion. In this moment, it's recommended to be honest in answering them. Prepare your mind to answer any questions and clear any doubts.

The subject will likely have questions both before or after the process has been completed. The primary reason for preparing is to build credibility and faith of your individual. If the subject is hesitant and distrustful of you, they is unlikely to be able to respond positively or follow your orders. The kinds of questions you're likely to receive and the possible responses you could give are listed below.

* Is this safe?

Absolutely. I am not going to alter your mind. You won't be compelled into saying or doing things you do not wish to. You are in control as I'll guide your steps. You will experience the focus and the precision of your subconscious. It will be a relaxing and a calming sensation. It's completely secure and once it's completed, you will return to the same person.

* What's your plan of course of

It's very easy. I'll ask you to comply with a few simple rules that you are expected to follow even if you're in a trance-like state. You are able to reject or refuse anything I tell you or request of you. You have the power to decide for your own thoughts and will be able to get out of the trance state on your own. I'll request you to think about or imagine some scenes and then have you narrate the things you're seeing in your eyes.

How does it feel to be in a state of hypnosis?

Hypnotism occurs when you are induced into an euphoric state. It is quite common, especially during sleep as dreams also have the capability of causing us to enter this state of trance. Hypnosis can help you concentrate your mind, provide clarity and ease your mind. It also improves your concentration and improves brain metabolism. It's similar to altering your mind when you are watching a wonderful television show or listen to an amazing piece of music. If you are absorbed and absorbed by something, you'll look at it from a different angle. For example, if you watch a film You become so immersed in it that you begin to see the film from a different angle rather than being part of the spectators. This is the way you feel when you are hypnotized.

* Can you force me to perform actions or make me do things I don't would

No. When you're hypnotized, however, you're still in control of your mind. Your personality , or mind isn't altered. You are able to reject any thing you would rather not do, and also not react if you aren't sure about what to say. You're in charge of yourself , and you shouldn't perform anything you wouldn't usually do.

* What are the ways I can become more attune?

The most efficient way you will be able to respond more effectively is to be relaxed. You'll be completely absorbed in your own thoughts. You'll be focused more intensely and exploring the potential in your mind. If you're willing to be a participant and you're keen to experience it , you'll respond more effectively. If you can focus and relax and relax and let the hypnotizer guide you, you'll be able be able to experience the effects of hypnotism more effectively.

* Could it be that there are situations in which I'm not interested in coming again?

The suggestions that a hypnotist will provide you with and the different instructions are exercises to help your mind. The goal is to delve deeper into your subconscious. You'll be in control of your thoughts and will be accountable to your decisions. When the hypnosis experience is finished, you will be more conscious and be back to your the normal level of consciousness. It's essentially an experience of deep relaxation. When this happens, it is possible that you will not wish to return but you won't be able to perform much while in the hypnotic condition. The hypnotizer also tries to get you back. It is also possible to be returned by yourself in situations of emergency.

* Are there instances where the hypnotist's method is not effective?

There are certain instances that hypnotism may take longer to take effect on certain people, but in general, everybody can be at ease. Imagine situations in which you are too absorbed in something you can't even hear what's going on in the surrounding area, or imagine an event in which you need to rise early and then be able to wake up the next morning. These are just a few examples that demonstrate that there are many abilities we have with our brains. It is incredibly powerful. A few of us have managed to improve our brains and then tune it into a specific way of thinking to go through our tasks. Most people who haven't previously hypnotized have a difficult experience getting hypnotized because of excitement, fear or other emotional states that don't allow them to relax completely. If you are able to focus and calm down and allow yourself to follow the hypnotizer's instructions, you'll be hypnotized a more quickly. If you actively participate and follow the directions of the hypnotizer, then you can achieve the success.

* If we are able to use our imagination when we do this what are the benefits?

Hypnotism is a method of channeling your imagination to focus and focus. It is a means of visualization and visualization. It helps your mind become more imaginative as it stimulates the brain and improves its efficiency. The brain is extremely strong because it is the control of every other body part, it's the organ that allows us to think, make decisions , and with proper training, we can increase our mental capacity. Hypnosis can help us achieve this.

Chapter 10: Self-Hypnosis

Self-hypnotism is a method to self-control. It can be employed to control your thoughts cravings, desires, urges and urges. Apart from the reasons mentioned above in the previous paragraph, it can also be employed to control your general mental state. Let's begin the journey with no further delay.

Like all good things that are able to be accessed in a series, self-hypnosis is one of three phases. It's not practical to begin any procedure on the wrong direction. This is why the procedure to induce self-hypnosis has been carefully broken down into three crucial steps. Starting with the beginning then we will look at how to prepare ourselves for the difficult process. The next stage will focus on the more concrete aspects in the procedure and the final stage will be concerned with the precautions and finalizing the actions that must be followed to be able to successfully conduct a self-hypnosis session.

Stage I - Preparation

The first part of your session must be as simple and basic as is possible. Simple beginnings always make sure that you don't off course from the primary purpose of the exercise. It is also a way to ensure that nothing overly complex is done in order to ensure that you remain focused and effective.

What are the best steps to follow to get yourself ready for self-hypnosis? Let's learn.

Clothing

Make sure that your clothes are not only simple, however they are also loose. It can be difficult to keep in your thoughts when the tight elastic of your new pajamas are causing blood loss. Instead of formals, or other clothing that hinders your blood flow, opt to something that resembles sweats or loose shorts.

Temperature

Find a setting that isn't too cold or hot. In a hot, humid atmosphere, you will cause you to sweat and thereby losing your water and causing you to be at risk of having too many water loss out of your body. A room that is extremely cold can affect you in the same way because the flow of blood and other vital organs of your body are affected. Choose a temperature that is at the middle between the extremes. You can make use of rooms heaters or air conditioners to control temperatures to match the temperature of the typical.

Place

After ensuring that the clothes you're wearing and the temperature you'll be working in are on the norm, it's now time to leave the location. Most often, the sessions are conducted inside, and self-hypnosis clients should choose an enclosed space for the process. Be sure that there isn't other person in the space you choose and close the door prior to starting the session. The room you choose must not be bright with regards to sunlight that comes from windows. Also, it is preferential that the room be slightly bent towards the dark aspect.

Posture

A single of the crucial aspects of hypnotism isn't what you or your partner sit, but rather how you are sitting. It goes without that the best place to hypnotize is sitting , not lying down. A lot of people have been reported to sleep as the session is going taking place, which is why we recommend to sit rather than lying down. Pick a couch or a chair to prepare yourself for the exercise. Make sure that none of your body has crossed particularly your legs and hands.

Aloneness

The main enemy to any hypnosis session would be disturbance. Be sure that prior to taking the position you are in on the chair that you turn off your mobile, close the windows and doors and shut down your computer and set your alarm clocks to a new time. Your hypnosis session will not be considered to have been successful in the event that you are interrupted by interruptions from your daily routine. If you're anticipating an urgent email or call, you must get rid of it prior to sitting down for the session. Keep in mind that this is the time of day that you set aside time for yourself. Nobody else, no matter how important, should be permitted to interrupt the sacred time of self-discovery.

Aims

It is essential to set an objective for your practice of hypnosis. Many people use it to eliminate undesirable habits, while some prefer to achieve calmness of the mind. Whatever your goal set your goals in your mind prior to before engaging in the self-hypnosis sessions. Setting goals is just as important as the achievement of those goals. If you don't have a specific objective in mind, then you'll be unable to focus on the solution which is meant to aid you.

The most popular motives for self-hypnosis are:

Stopping bad habits, people drink or smoke, and gamble! Many undesirable behaviors can be found among the populace. To eliminate these habits, you can use self-hypnosis.

The peace of mind is the most sought-after objective in our modern world. Our lives are too hectic and complex that stress and mental angst will surely affect our mental stability. In such a situation, it is essential to find a way to attain some form of mental peace. Self-hypnosis can be the solution.

A few people wish to enhance their brain's performance. The brain functions similar to a puppy. If you train it right from the beginning it will be able to learn quickly and pay attention to your instructions. Training your brain is as crucial as everything else. Self-hypnosis is an excellent method to gain access to the amazing power of control of the brain.

Your mind is an effective tool. If you use it wisely it will produce great outcomes. Its health will determine your character and outlook on the world. The overall progress of your life is contingent on how well your mind responds and runs. Self-hypnosis can help keep your mind focus and sharp throughout the day, giving you to achieve self-improvement, without meditation or yoga classes.

The initial stage of self-hypnosis is to prepare yourself as well as your mind and body, for the lengthy self-hypnosis process. This phase is not to be taken lightly as it could result in a drastic backfiring. It's all about building your structure starting from the first brick. Be sure to build your foundations sturdy and have the foundations are correct.

After we've mastered the basics, we are able to move on.

Close your eyes

Closing your eyes can have an uplifting effect on your eyes. It will be apparent you have eyes that are most efficient aspect of your sensory system. Your eyes allow you to be aware of the world around you. If you close your eyes around fifty percent of the disturbance you could have received has dispersed to other areas. The first step in any kind of meditation activity is to shut your eyes. This is not just a way to regulate the flow of light, but it also stops any visual distraction from entering your thoughts.

Take your thoughts off the table

The most crucial element of this phase and the entire experience is this. Once you get started, you'll be aware that despite your attempts to grin and smirk but you're not able to get out of your mind; that even though you do your best at it, some random thoughts continue to wander around your head like all the thoughts of the world are conspiring against your mental absence. It's normal. Do not be afraid because you're not able to completely eliminate thoughts. Try your best at first. If you fail, do it again. It is not easy for everyone to succeed in such things on their first try.

Be Impartial

The best method to stop thinking thoughts to not enter into your head is to be an objective observer and not a passionate judge. Recognize how much you respond to thoughts the more they'll bother your mind by repeating them in your head. The best way to deal with this is to sit still and take a step back and observe your thoughts, without making one single comment about their nature. If, for instance, it thoughts come to mind the desire to savor a delicious pizza, just forget about it. You must have eaten your meal prior to the time to ensure that a thought won't affect your eating habits in any way. This is known as impartiality, which is a useful technique to stop thoughts from affecting.

An Alternative

If you're struggling to not think about it, build a pontoon for the opposite wall and concentrate your thoughts on it. It does not have to be a line; it could be a smudge , too. All you need is a well-focused center of interest and you're good go.

Stage II: Play the Tension

Find the tensions in your body. To find the tension it is necessary to segregate every body part from the other , and then feel tension in every body part in a different way. Start with the toes because they are the lower the body part. Concentrate on the area you are focusing on and notice when the tension begins to ease off. Make use of your imagination to imagine the tension moving through your feet, toes and calves, your the chest, stomach and head away from your surroundings. Relax the tension slowly but gradually. Don't rush this process since it might cause harm to the goal of it.

Breathes

Another crucial stepto take is breathing. It can do amazing for your health and make a significant contributions to your self-hypnosis sessions. As you breath, the lungs expand and relax, providing sufficient body heat and fitness to continue. When you are in a self-hypnosis program it is crucial to let yourself relax. Relax and take deep, slow breaths. Each breath that you take, you'll observe positive energy entering your body. Every exhalation will make you realize the negativity that has left your body. It is possible to use with your imagination to create your visual image. Imagine the intake of air as a bright ball of sun and the air that is emitted as a dark, gloomy cloud that hovers over a village that is in need of help; treating its crops to ruin.

Imagine:

If you're close to being enticed by self-hypnosis it's about time to begin falling further into the labyrinths that are the mind of your imagination. Consider imagining yourself on top of your most cherished tower. It is impossible to see below you but the vast expanse of space. Then there is water. Imagine that you've received a pair of wings, but you've never been on a flight before, and you're hesitant about going down. Relax and do an unintentional risk. Imagine falling in the air for the first time in your life. This is the moment of your liberation.

Visualize every single detail of the scene with your imagination. Make an effort to go into the deepest details. Are your wings pale, flimsy and brown or black like raven's wings; sturdy and solid? Change your appearance and leap, without fear anywhere in the world.

Get deeper

You've now made the leap. There's of course there is no way back. It is the time to moved on to the next phase, which is the best place to explore your thoughts. The pool of water you could see in the top part of your head tower is now threatening to reach your. It's not gravity pushing you there; you're all by yourself. Take a look! You're flying!

Do you feel that floating sensation? Now, you're supposed to feel more light than you did before. Gravity has stopped working against you, instead there is a form of gravity that only you can control. As time passes, you become the control of your own actions. Then you begin floating, but your wings are in your control.

Say

We are at an era where a real game might be launched. Choose one statement. The statement should be based on your goals. For instance, you might want to end a bad habit, such as smoking. It could be something like "I'm going quit smoking. Then Try to make it as simple as you can and incorporate the idea into your brain's awareness.

Once you've achieved the above mentioned sensation of floating and you feel comfortable, you can repeat the phrase in loops. Use a soft but robust tone repeat the phrase five times within minutes, leaving breaks in between. Once you've got the hang of it, consider increasing the frequency, and repeat it ten, then twenty times within a minute. Continue this process until you reach the number of thirty.

Walk out

Make sure you never get out of a self-hypnosis state. If you decide suddenly to snap right out of of hypnosis, it may cause harm to you mental wellbeing in a variety of extreme ways. To stop your self-hypnosis, just go back to where you left off. As I recall you were flying. Slowly descend until you reach the building you flew over. Take the wings off your arms, and then walk through the stairs. Be sure to walk with a steady pace in case you fall. Accidents that happen in your mind can have a negative impact on your the real world too. A seamless transition from hypnosis to reality is preferable to the shock of a sudden snapping.

Stage III: Enhancement

The self-hypnosis process will not perform if you don't have the determination to make changes or take charge of your life. Keep in mind that hypnosis is just an instrument, and you are the main person. Every morning, you must repeat your words before the mirror. Do not allow yourself to be enticed by the urges you promised you wouldn't be attracted through your daily routine. Get rid of the bad habits that you said you would.

After waking up to terms with reality that you adhere to the promises you made when you were under hypnosis. Utilize you imagination in order to make yourself feel more confident about yourself. Whatever goal you're trying to reach, visualize yourself achieving it. Develop the confidence in yourself and the mental courage within you to push more hard towards achieving the objective that you have set.

Chapter 11: Sample Hypnotic Scripts

The key to hypnotizing individuals, whether they are you or someone else it is to use the correct words in the correct way. This chapter I will present to you a variety of scripts to hypnotize in various scenarios which you can use either as they are or in a modified form. If you'd like to perform self-hypnosis yourself, you can record yourself speaking these scripts and then listen to them at a suitable time.

For hypnotic scripts from 2 to 19, you can use the induction, deepening , and awakening scripts of Script #1 to bring the subject into a state of hypnosis take them further into the trance and, following the scripts as a suggestions, help them get out, if desired.

Script #1: General Hypnosis

Induction (to induce subject to a state of Trance)

Then, you will experience a heightened sleep-inducing sensation. But, if you might need to be awakened by circumstances that require and urgent, there is no problem doing so due to the alertness and possibilities. It is possible that you require an extremely comfortable posture, relax and close your eyes. This can provide a sense of comfort. There is nothing to do. The most important thing is to concentrate on breathing and exhaling. Keep your focus on inhalation and eventually release it slowly to relax.

Continue to work to develop a sequence of slow inhalation and exhalation, then exhaling slowly. Continue to work in this manner.

As you move through the process, you'll think that you're healthy and in good shape.

There is no need to be doing or possessing anything unique or be in a particular location to be able to go on the hypnotic stage. Recall good memories and positive feelings while you are on another stage that is hypnotic.

Allow this course of action to unfold take your thoughts out of you and take in the sensations of what's going on in your body. Allow it to flow until it responds to the words.

Remember and understand every action that was taken in reaction to my words. how wonderful and perfect the understanding is.

Imagine your breathing patterns flowing through your solar plexus. Then, imagine colors that will allow you to relax and ease in this moment. Let these colors flow within you, throughout your entire body, beginning from your head to your toes.

Relax your muscles and let them relax, turn soft and observe the reaction of your body that gives an additional feeling of joy as well as a pleasurable and comfortable sensation that will leave you feeling completely.

When this happens you can feel the connection between your body and mind , where your mind is listening and continues to follow.

In this thrilling experience the only thing you can do is keep in your mind the good memories, thoughts and images. The mind guides you to the place where the body is at the present moment.

Deepening

Then, I'd like to see the wall from the perspective of your brain. When you complete the process, you're likely to notice all the figures from 20 to 1 falling down one at a time onto the wall. You will be able to remember them as striking and cooperative as I begin to talk about the 20th number going down to 1.

The numbers you are seeing are no longer in order due to my counting down to the number 1. The number decreases in size. When I get to the number 15 it is possible to believe that the numbers have disappeared when they get shrinking and becoming smaller. In this time you're in the most intense and revealing experience.